THE MOVEMENT SYSTEM

Athlete Upper Quarter

JARED VAGY PT, DPT, OCS, CSCS
Doctor of Physical Therapy
Board Certified Clinical Specialist

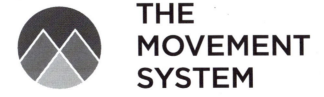

themovementsystem@gmail.com
athletemovementsytem.com
@athletemovementsystem

The Movement System Foundational Assessment

The Application of Foundational Concepts in the UQ

Jared Vagy PT, DPT, OCS, CSCS

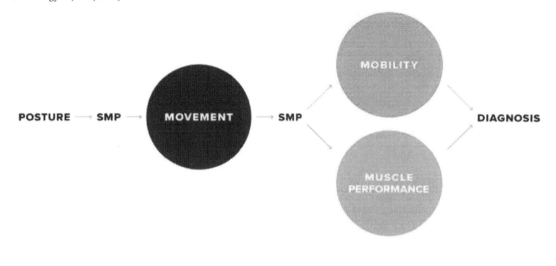

SMP = Symptom Modification Procedure

Course Schedule Day 1

- **8am-9am:** Lecture: Introduction and foundational assessment
- **9am-11am:** Lecture: Foundational assessment techniques
- **11am-12pm:** Lab: Foundational assessment techniques
- **12-1PM:** Lunch
- **1-2PM:** Lecture: Biomechanics and advanced assessment
- **2-5PM:** Lab: Advanced assessment techniques

Course Objectives

- Understand the importance of regional interdependence of the upper quarter and its functional relationship to pathobiomechanics.

- Learn the 4 foundational and 5 advanced movement science concepts.

- Identify the key critical events of the described sports and select appropriate movement assessments for the upper quarter.

- Provide interventions based on a rehabilitation pyramid by linking the key movement impairments from the objective examination to the critical event of the specific sport.

Copyright © 2019 Dr. Jared Vagy DPT

About the Instructor

Jared Vagy PT, DPT, OCS, CSCS

- Doctor of Physical Therapy
- Orthopedic Clinical Specialist
- Residency Training: Orthopedics
- Fellowship Training: Movement Science
- Adjunct Instructor of Clinical Physical Therapy at USC
- Orthopedic Residency Mentor
- Numerous publications on injury prevention
- Chinese National Team Track & Field Summer 2015, Team USA Olympic Team Track and Field Trials 2016, US Olympic Training Committee Sports Medicine Rotation 2017
- Editorial Board of Advance Rehab Magazine
- OCS test item writer

Copyright © 2019 Dr. Jared Vagy DPT

Special Thanks

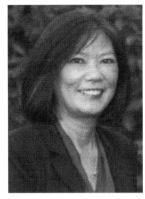 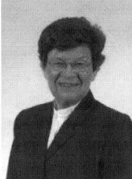 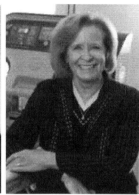 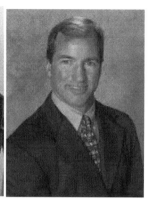

Clare Frank   Shirley Sahrmann   Beth Fisher   Chris Powers

Special Thanks

USC Division of Biokinesiology and Physical Therapy

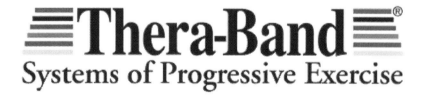
Systems of Progressive Exercise

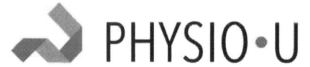
TOP RATED CLINICAL REASONING SOFTWARE AT YOUR FINGERTIPS

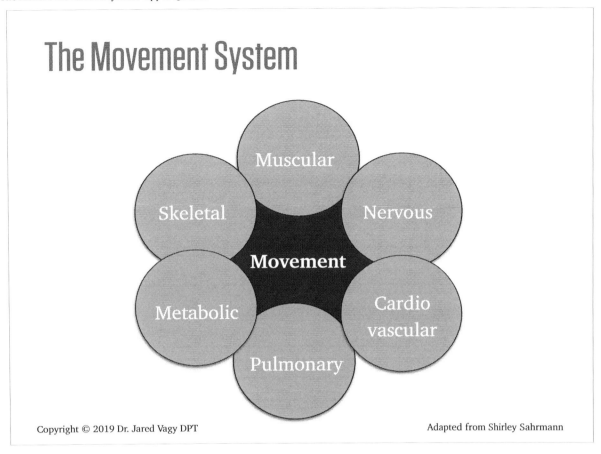

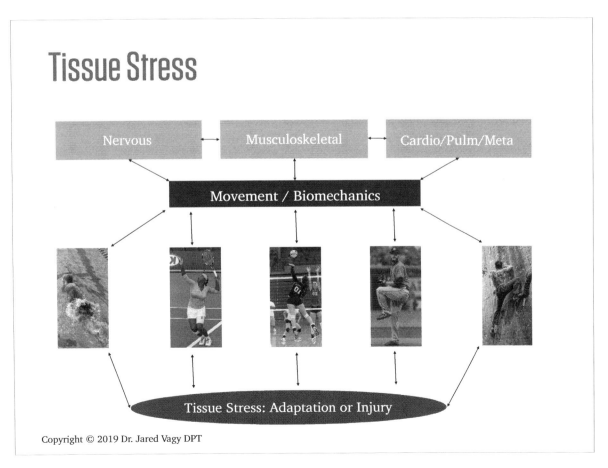

Introduction to Upper Quarter Injury

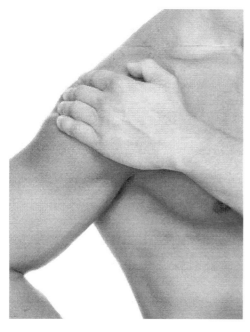

- World wide, cost of sports injuries:
  $1 Billion annually (Eger 1990)

- Americans who receive medical attention for sports-related injuries:
  $7 Million annually (Conn et al 2003)

Upper Extremity vs. Lower Extremity

- More attention is given to lower extremity sports injuries in comparison to upper extremity injuries.

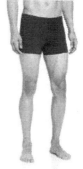

- The ankle and knee are the most frequently injured body regions. (Burt et al 2001)

- Upper extremity injuries account for 35% of all sports injuries. (Sytema 2010)

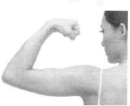

Types of Injury

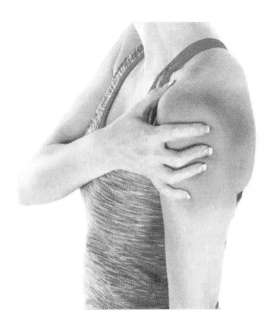

- **Acute:** Direct trauma or sudden overload of tissue.

- **Chronic:** Overuse injury, repeated cumulative microtrauma.

- **Acute on chronic:** Sudden rupture of previously damaged tissue.

Copyright © 2019 Dr. Jared Vagy DPT

Prevalence of Upper Extremity Injury

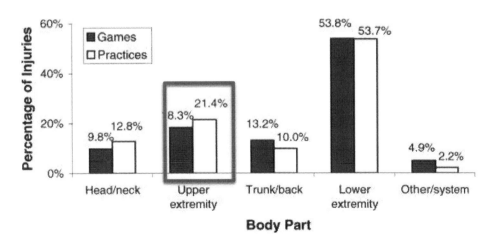

Distribution in % of injuries by body part for games and practices for 15 sports, National Collegiate Athletic Association, 1988–1989 through 2003–2004 (Hootman et al 2007)

Copyright © 2019 Dr. Jared Vagy DPT

Prevalence Increases with Age

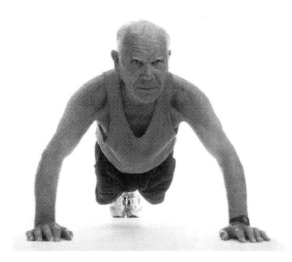

- Prevalence of shoulder pain increases with age. (Van der Windt 1999)

- Shoulder complaints increase with age, peaking in the 40–49 and 50–59 year age brackets. (Bot et al 2005)

Tissue Healing Time

Table 4. Healing Rates of Tissues.*

	0–3 days	4–14 days	3–4 weeks	5–7 weeks	2–3 months	3–6 months	6 months –1 year	Up to 2 years
Tendon								
• Tendinitis			←—→	←———→				
• Lacerations				←———→	←———→	←———→		
Muscle								
• Exercise-induced	←—→							
• Grade I	←———→	←———→						
• Grade II		←———→	←———→	←———→	←———→			
• Grade III			←———→	←———→	←———→	←———→		
Ligament								
• Grade I	←—→							
• Grade II			←———→	←———→	←———→			
• Grade III				←———→	←———→	←———→	←———→	
Ligament Graft					←———→	←———→	←———→	←———→
Bone				←———→	←———→			
Articular Cartilage Repair					←———→	←———→	←———→	←———→

(Axe et al 2005)

Overhead Sports

- Swimming *ave 30,000 revolutions/wk !*
    - 38-75% of competitive swimmers reported shoulder pain. (McMaster 1993)
- Tennis
    - Shoulder pain increased to 50% in middle-aged tennis players. (Lehman 1988)
    - 31-51% of recreational players will have tennis elbow. (De Smedt et al. 2007)
- Volleyball
    - Shoulder pain is the second most common overuse-related condition, accounting for 8–20% of all volleyball injuries. (Verhagen 2004)
- Baseball
    - Roughly half of youth pitchers reported elbow or shoulder pain during the season. (Lyman 2002)
- Rock Climbing
    - Overuse injuries accounting for 93% of all injuries (Backe et al. 2009) 40 percent fingers, 16 percent shoulders, 12 percent elbows, 5 percent knees, 5 percent back and 4 percent wrists. (Reay et al 2000)

Copyright © 2019 Dr. Jared Vagy DPT

4 Foundational Concepts

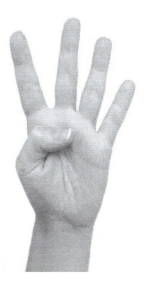

1. The Movement System
    - Scapular, humeral and thoracic assessment
2. Joint Centration
    - Path of instantaneous center of rotation
3. Relative Flexibility ← *TB tension example.*
    - Short versus relative stiffness
4. Muscle Performance
    - The quality, timing and MVIC of a muscle contraction

Copyright © 2019 Dr. Jared Vagy DPT

Symptom Modification Procedures

- A alternative method of treatment based clinical examination
- A series of four mechanical techniques that are applied while the patient performs the activity or movement that most closely reproduces the symptoms experienced by the patient
- Humeral, scapular, cervico/thoracic and thoracic tests are described

Symptom modification procedures can be used to guide treatment based clinical decisions. Clinical reasoning is applied to pain alleviating techniques as opposed to pain provoking special tests that lack diagnostic accuracy.

[margin note: alleviating vs. aggravation (special tests)]

Lewis, J. S. (2009) Rotator cuff tendinopathy/subacromial impingement syndrome: is it time for a new method of assessment? British Journal of Sports Medicine, Vol 43, pp. 259-264

The Movement System

POSTURE → SMP → MOVEMENT → SMP → MOBILITY / MUSCLE PERFORMANCE → DIAGNOSIS

SMP = Symptom Modification Procedure

Posture

Posterior	Lateral	Anterior
Cervical • Creasing, sidebend or rotation	Cervical • Ear in line with shoulder • Chin angle 90 deg	Cervical • Accessory muscle hypertrophy
Scapula Position • T2-T7 • Elevation/depression • 3" from midline • 3-10 deg anterior tilt	Thoracic spine • Excessive kyphosis/ straightening	Clavicle angle • 20 deg inclined Rib angle • 90 degrees
Humerus • Olecranon rotation • Arm windows	Humerus • Flex/Ext • Anterior Glide	Humerus • Cubital fossa crease

SA kicks in @ 60°

Tyler test?

Movement

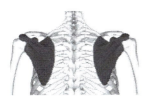
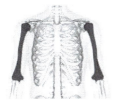
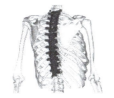

Scapular Faults
- Excessive winging/medial rotation
- Insufficient posterior tipping
- Insufficient upward rotation and elevation

Humeral Faults
- Excessive humeral anterior translation
- Excessive humeral medial rotation

Thoracic Faults
- Insufficient thoracic extension

Joint Centration

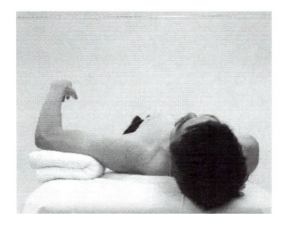

Centrated Joint

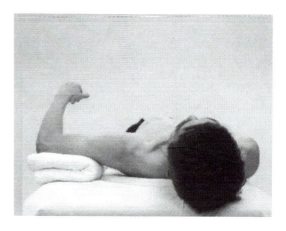

Non-centrated Joint

Copyright © 2019 Dr. Jared Vagy DPT

Relative Flexibility

PROM
SH ✓
Muscle w/ mobility deficit

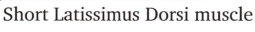

Short Latissimus Dorsi muscle   Black - Black = stretch!

Relative stiffness of the Latissimus Dorsi muscle

Copyright © 2019 Dr. Jared Vagy DPT

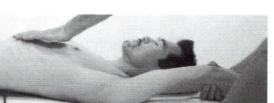

Yellow — Black ← use relaxation tech. to change to yellow.
↑
stiffen
"core strengthening"

Muscular Performance

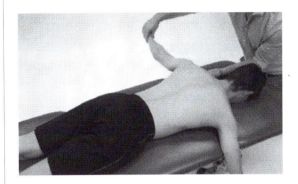 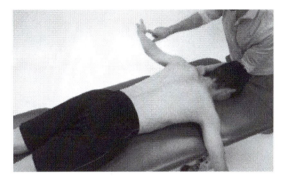

5/5 Mid Trapezius Muscle Test without Compensation

5/5 Mid Trapezius Muscle Test with Compensation

Research: Manual Muscle Testing

- 53 participants with unilateral shoulder pain
- Performed 3 manual muscle strength assessments to determine weakness between involved and uninvolved shoulders Assessments performed twice
    - Using manual resistance grading
    - Hand-held dynamometry
- Found that muscle weakness in injured shoulder compared to the opposite (uninvolved shoulder) could not be detected among patients with 60-99% strength of uninvolved shoulder

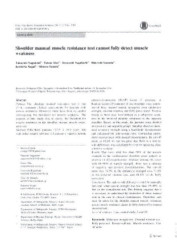

Patient can have up to 60% strength difference on one side and not be detectable

Nagatomi T, et al. "Shoulder manual muscle resistance test cannot fully detect muscle weakness." *Knee Surg Sports Traumatol Arthrosc.* 2017;25:2081-2088.

Research: Hand-Held Dynamometry

- A sample of 106 men and 125 women volunteers were tested twice with an Ametek digital hand-held dynamometer.
- The measurements were found to be reliable.
- Predictive equations were provided for the measurements.
- Reference values generated are expressed in Newtons and as a percentage of body weight and are organized by gender, decade of age, and side.

Hand-held dynamometry is a reliable assessment and values obtained in a clinical setting can determine if an individual is impaired relative to healthy subjects of the same gender and age.

Bohannon, Richard W. "Reference values for extremity muscle strength obtained by hand-held dynamometry from adults aged 20 to 79 years." Archives of physical medicine and rehabilitation 78.1 (1997): 26-32.

Is the Difference Worth the Cost?

Luggage Scale	Grip Dynamometer	Crane Scale	Dynamometer
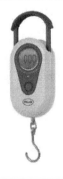	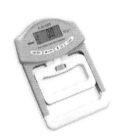	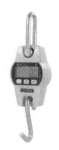	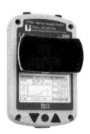
$10	$25	$50	$1000

- 0-44 lbs
- Continuous force

- 0-200 lbs
- Peak force
- Fixed test time

- 0-600 lbs
- Peak force
- Fixed test time

- 0-300 lbs
- Peak force
- Time to reach peak force
- Variable total test time
- Average force

Copyright © 2017 Dr. Jared Vagy DPT

Dynamometer Testing

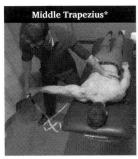
Middle Trapezius*

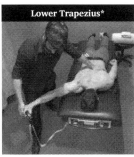
Lower Trapezius*

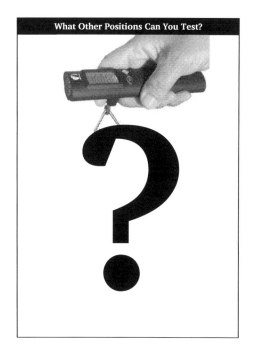
What Other Positions Can You Test?

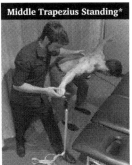
Middle Trapezius Standing*

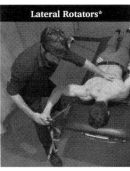
Lateral Rotators*

Copyright © 2017 Dr. Jared Vagy DPT   * The style of the dynamometer will dictate the hand position.

Integration of the Movement System

Scapular Faults
- Excessive winging/medial rotation
- Insufficient posterior tipping
- Insufficient upward rotation and elevation

Humeral Faults
- Excessive humeral anterior translation
- Excessive humeral medial rotation

Thoracic Faults
- Insufficient thoracic extension

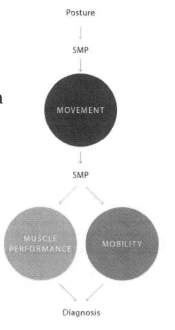

Excessive Scapular Winging and IR

Posture Observation	Excessive scapular winging and medial rotation
Posture SMP	Scapular adduction and ER reposition
Movement Observation	Excessive scapular winging and medial rotation with shoulder flexion and abduction
Movement SMP	Scapular protraction resistance cue past 60 deg Scapular adduction and ER reposition
Mobility	Pec Minor Posterior Rotator Cuff
Muscle Performance	Serratus Anterior Middle Trapezius Rhomboid

Excessive Scapular Winging and IR

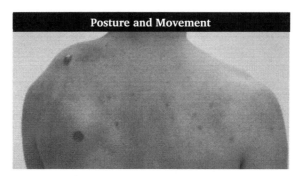
Posture and Movement

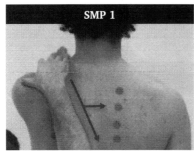
SMP 1

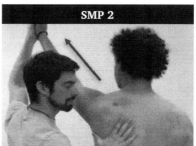
SMP 2

SMP Posture

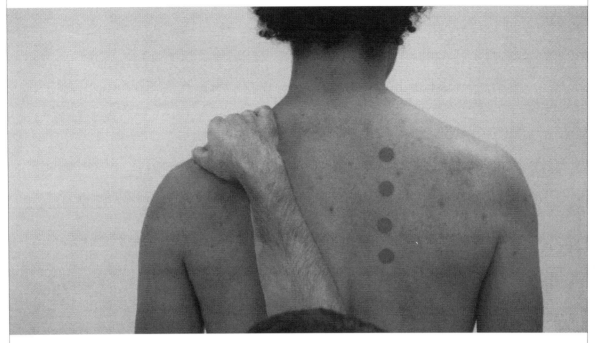

SMP Movement

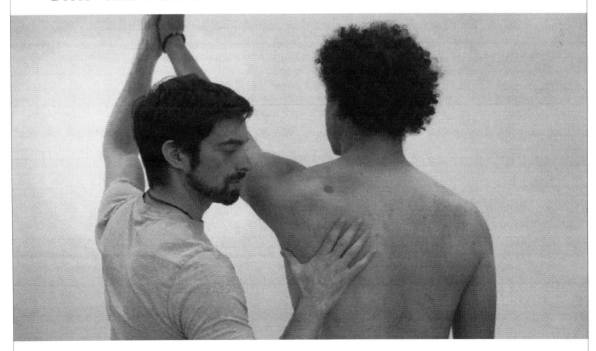

Research: Scapular Stability

- 142 Division 1 Overhead Athletes
- Performed 3 Shoulder Impingement Assessments and measured Isometric elevation strength
    - Scapula in natural resting position
    - Scapula Reposition Test position
- 47% of athletes who reported pain with Impingement assessments had significant pain reduction with Scapula Reposition Test
- 55% of athletes had significant strength gains with Scapula Reposition Test

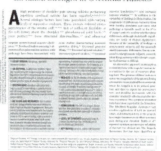

Manually repositioning the scapula, using the scapula reposition test, yields increased elevation strength and decreased pain in over-head athletes.

Lawrence R, Braman J, Laprade R, Ludewig P. Comparison of 3-Dimensional Shoulder Complex Kinematics in Individuals with and without Shoulder Pain, Part 1: SC, AC, and ST Joints. JOSPT 2014. 44(9) 636-A8

Insufficient Scapular Posterior Tipping

Posture Observation	Excessive scapular anterior tipping
Posture SMP	Scapular assist with posterior tip
Movement Observation	Insufficient scapular posterior tipping with shoulder flexion and abduction
Movement SMP	Scapular assist with posterior tip
Mobility	Pec Minor
Muscle Performance	Lower Trapezius

Research: Posterior Tipping

- 22 participants (10 shoulder impingement, 12 control) underwent 3-D movement analysis of shoulder flexion, abduction, and scaption.
- Subjects were asked to lift arms into flexion, scaption, and abduction.
- Difference in scapulothoracic, acromioclavicular, and sternocostal kinematics were recorded.

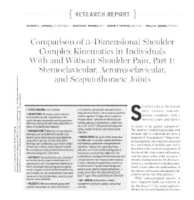

Those with shoulder impingement demonstrated significantly less scapular upward rotation and sternoclavicular posterior rotation

Lawrence R, Braman J, Laprade R, Ludewig P. Comparison of 3-Dimensional Shoulder Complex Kinematics in Individuals with and without Shoulder Pain, Part 1: SC, AC, and ST Joints. JOSPT 2014. 44(9) 636-A8

Insufficient Scapular Posterior Tipping

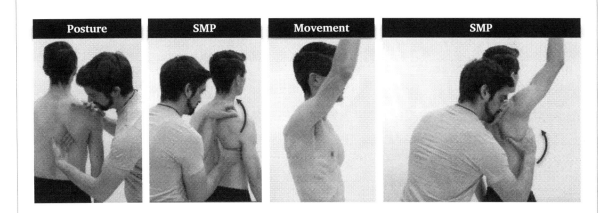

Copyright © 2019 Dr. Jared Vagy DPT

SMP Posture

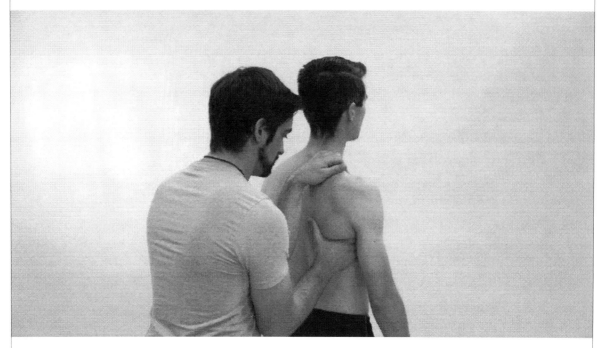

SMP Movement

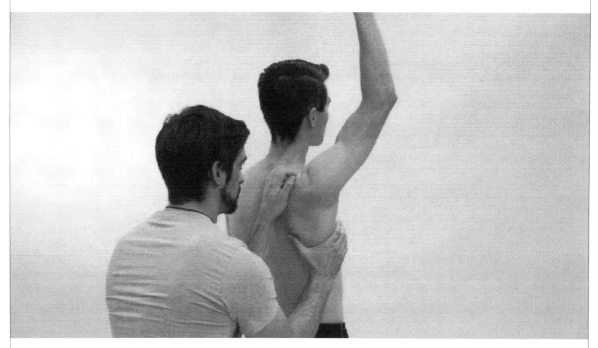

Insufficient Scapular Upward Rot/Elevation

Posture Observation	Scapular Downward Rotation Scapular Depression
Posture SMP	Scapular assist upward rotation Scapular assist elevation
Movement Observation	Insufficient scapular upward rotation and elevation with shoulder flexion or abduction
Movement SMP	Scapular assist upward rotation Scapular assist elevation
Mobility	Levator Scapula Rhomboids Latissimus Dorsi
Muscle Performance	Upper Trapezius Lower Trapezius Serratus Anterior

Copyright © 2019 Dr. Jared Vagy DPT

Research: Upward Rotation

- 46 adolescent swimmers and 43 adolescent non-swimmers were measured in 4 positions: neutral, hands on hips, 90° abduction, and full abduction
- Measurements of: superior angle to spine, inferior angle to spine, anterior humeral head to anterior acromion, and BMI were measured.
- 12 month follow up to determine incidence of shoulder pain

Patients with shorter distances between the scapula and the spine, indicating decreased scapular upward rotation, were more likely to develop shoulder pain

McKenna L, Straker L, Smith A, Can Scapular and Humeral Head Position Predict Shoulder Pain in Adolescent Swimmers and Non-Swimmers? Journal of Sports Sciences, 2012. 30(16) 1767-1776.

Insufficient Scapular Upward Rot/Elevation

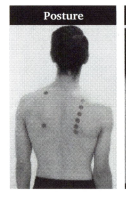 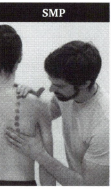 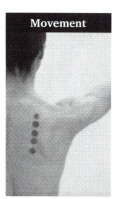 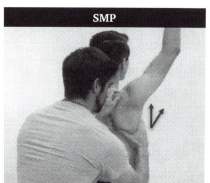

upper trap resting pain

SMP Posture

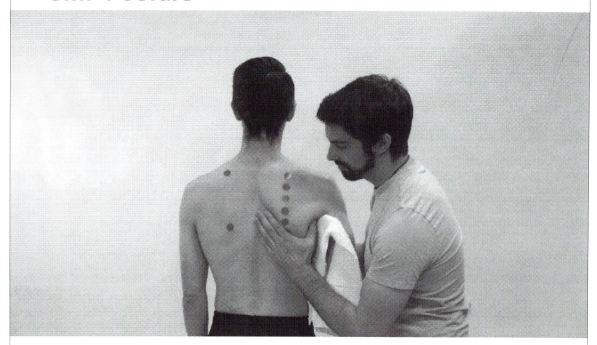

SMP Movement

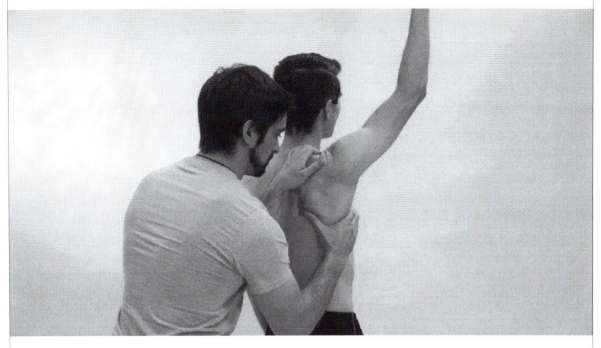

Excessive Humeral Anterior Translation

upper trap pain and rotating

Posture Observation	Excessive humeral anterior translation
Posture SMP	Posterior glide standing
Movement Observation	Excessive humeral anterior translation with shoulder flexion, abduction and medial rotation
Movement SMP	Posterior glide standing during flexion/abduction Posterior glide supine during medial rotation
Mobility	Posterior glenohumeral joint capsule Posterior Rotator Cuff
Muscle Performance	Posterior Rotator Cuff ← strengthen eccentrically!! Subscapularis ← This is joint centering

— Tyler's test to differentiate

(teres Major, Pec are not)

Research: Humeral Anterior Translation

- Three 1st division handball players with dysfunction in late cocking phase were compared to age-matched non-athlete controls with high speed CT scan and 3-D reconstruction.
- Arthrokinematic position of the humerus on the glenoid in 90/90 and late cocking phase were compared, with rotation and translation.

Participants with micro instability showed increased superior and anterior migration of the humeral head during late cocking

Baeyens, J. P., Van Roy, P., De Schepper, A., Declercq, G., & Clarijs, J. P. (2001). Glenohumeral joint kinematics related to minor anterior instability of the shoulder at the end of the late preparatory phase of throwing. *Clinical Biomechanics*, 16(9), 752–757. http://doi.org/10.1016/S0268-0033(01)00068-7

Excessive Humeral Anterior Translation

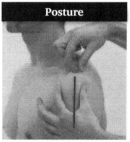
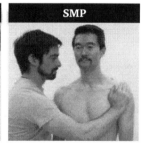
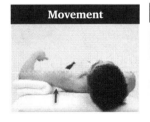
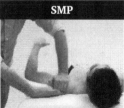
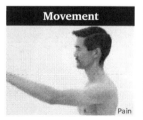
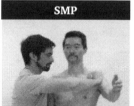

Copyright © 2019 Dr. Jared Vagy DPT

SMP Movement

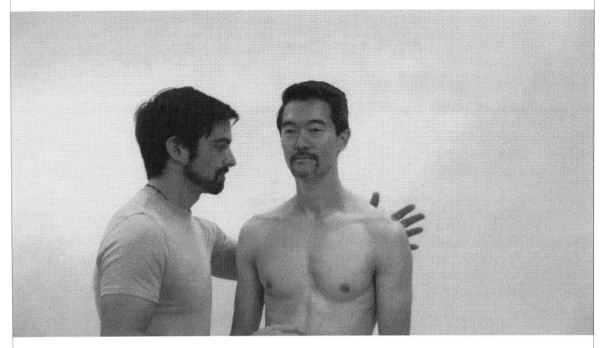

SMP Movement

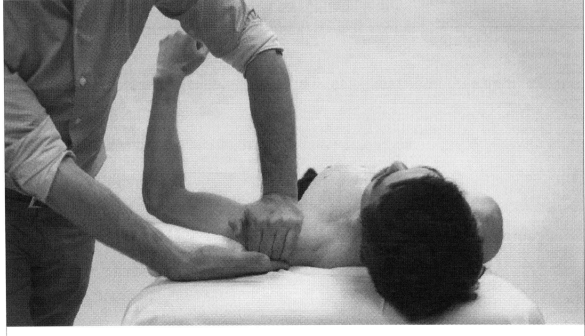

Excessive Humeral Medial Rotation

(handwritten: ① anterior or posterior SH)

Posture Observation	Excessive humeral medial rotation
Posture SMP	Humeral lateral rotation
Movement Observation	Excessive humeral medial rotation with shoulder flexion and abduction
Movement SMP	Humeral lateral rotation
Mobility	Subscapularis Pec Major Latissimus Dorsi Teres Major
Muscle Performance	Infraspinatus Teres Minor

Copyright © 2019 Dr. Jared Vagy DPT

Research: Excessive Humeral Medial Rotation

- 22 participants (10 shoulder impingement, 12 control) underwent 3-D movement analysis of shoulder flexion, abduction, and scaption.
- Subjects were asked to lift arms into flexion, scaption, and abduction.
- Difference glenohumeral joint motion was monitored

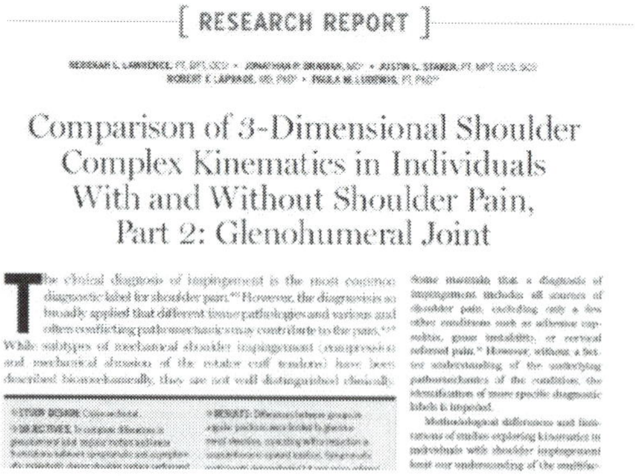

Subjects with shoulder impingement demonstrated less postural glenohumeral joint external rotation when compared to controls

Lawrence, R. L., Braman, J. P., Staker, J. L., Laprade, R. F., & Ludewig, P. M. (2014). Comparison of 3-Dimensional Shoulder Complex Kinematics in Individuals With and Without Shoulder Pain, Part 2: Glenohumeral Joint. Journal of Orthopaedic & Sports Physical Therapy, 44(9), 646-B3. http://doi.org/10.2519/jospt.2014.5556

Excessive Humeral Medial Rotation

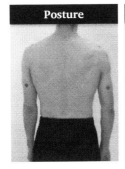
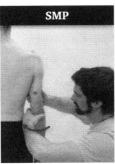
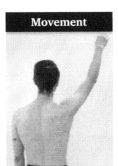
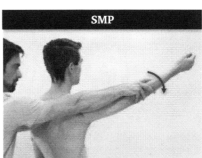

SMP Posture

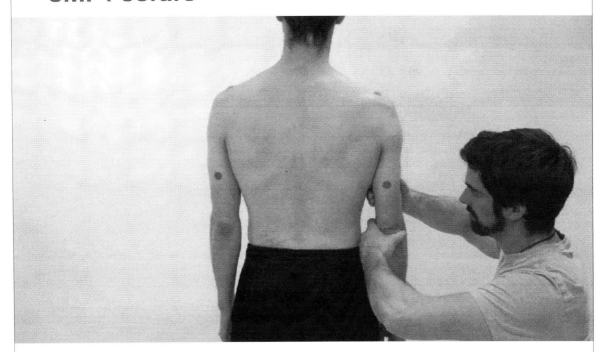

SMP Movement

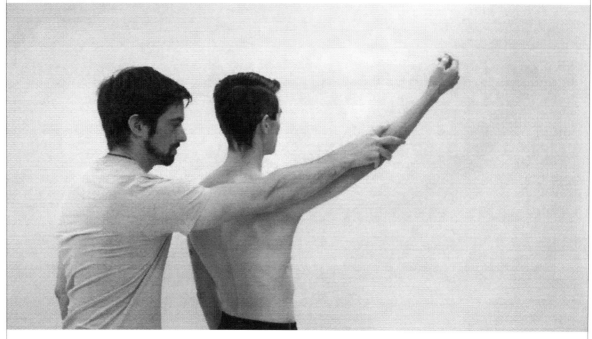

Insufficient Thoracic Extension

Posture Observation	Thoracic Kyphosis
Posture SMP	Thoracic extension facilitation
Movement Observation	Insufficient thoracic extension with shoulder flexion
Movement SMP	Thoracic extension facilitation
Mobility	Thoracic spinal accessory mobility
Muscle Performance	Paraspinals Multifidi Lower Trapezius Middle Trapezius

Research: Insufficient Thoracic Extension

- 2144 participants were followed at routine physicals for incidence of shoulder pain.
- All subjects also were tested using: wall occiput test (WOT), and rib-pelvic-distance-test, UE quick dash, and Neer and Hawkins-Kennedy.
- Positive WOT is indicative of increased thoracic kyphosis

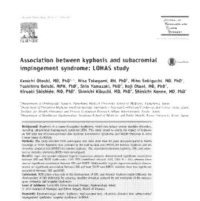

Significantly more participants with thoracic kyphosis developed shoulder pain than those who did not have thoracic kyphosis

Otoshi, K., Takegami, M., Sekiguchi, M., Onishi, Y., Yamazaki, S., Otani, K., ... Konno, S. (2014). Association between kyphosis and subacromial impingement syndrome: LOHAS study. Journal of Shoulder and Elbow Surgery, 23(12), e300–e307. http://doi.org/10.1016/j.jse.2014.04.010

Insufficient Thoracic Extension

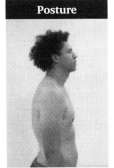
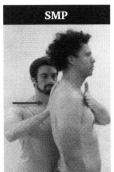
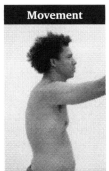
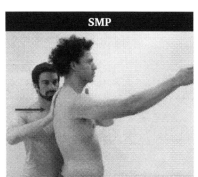

Copyright © 2019 Dr. Jared Vagy DPT

SMP Posture

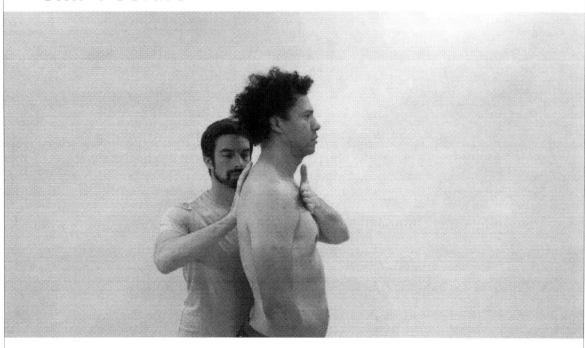

SMP Movement

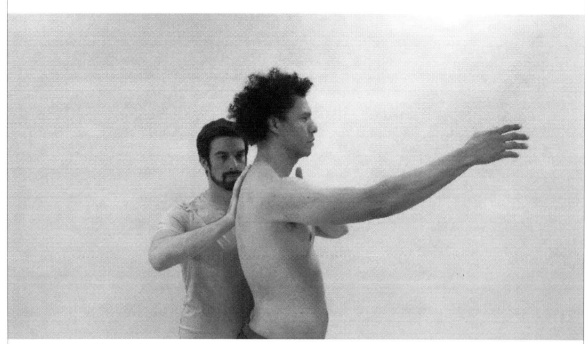

Summary

1. The Movement System
   - Scapular, humeral and thoracic assessment
2. Joint Centration
   - Path of instantaneous center of rotation
3. Relative Flexibility
   - Short versus relative stiffness
4. Muscle Performance
   - The quality, timing and MVIC of a muscle contraction

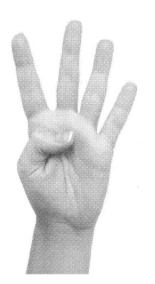

Copyright © 2019 Dr. Jared Vagy DPT

Biomechanics and Advanced Assessment

The Application of Advanced Concepts in the UQ

Jared Vagy PT, DPT, OCS, CSCS

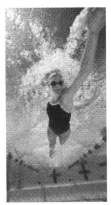 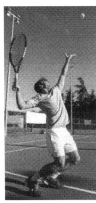 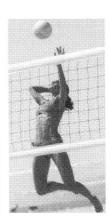 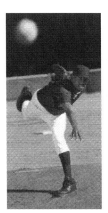 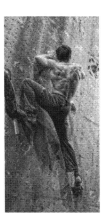

Copyright © 2017 Dr. Jared Vagy DPT

5 Advanced Concepts

1. **Mirroring Movement** (Climbing)
2. **Video Analysis** (Baseball)
3. **Dysfunctional Position** (Swimming)
4. **Kinetic Chain** (Tennis)
5. **Critical Events** (Volleyball)

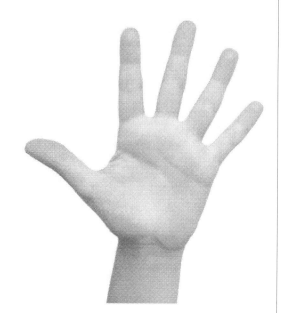

Mirroring Movement

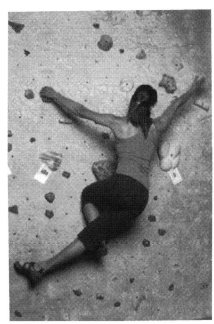
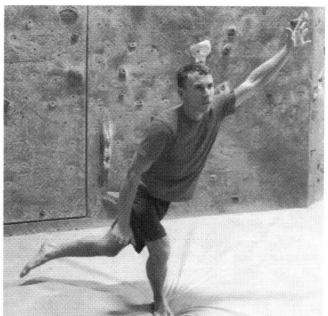

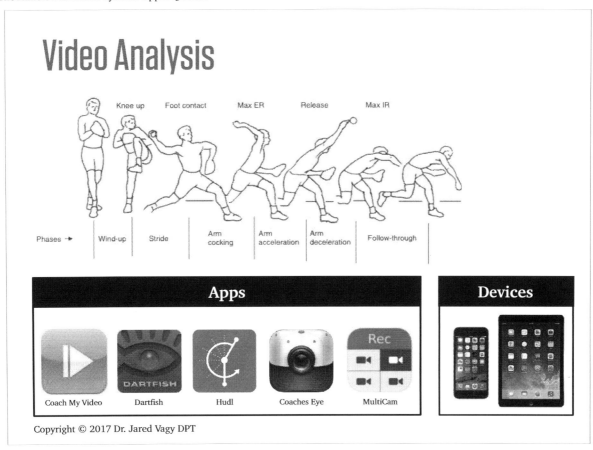

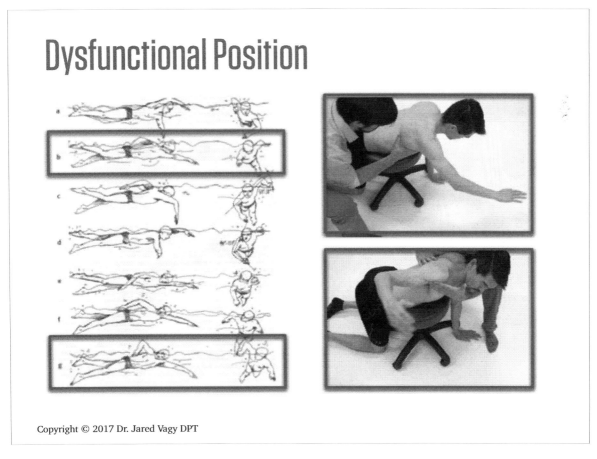

Kinetic Chain

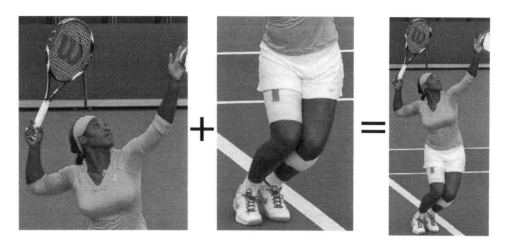

It is essential to assess and treat the entire kinetic chain. If you don't analyze movement, you are missing a large piece of the puzzle.

Critical Events

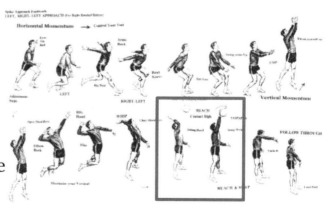

✓ Wind Up Phase
✓ Cocking Phase
✓ Acceleration Phase
  ✓ Ball Contact
✓ Deceleration Phase
✓ Follow Through Phase

Copyright © 2017 Dr. Jared Vagy DPT

Climbing

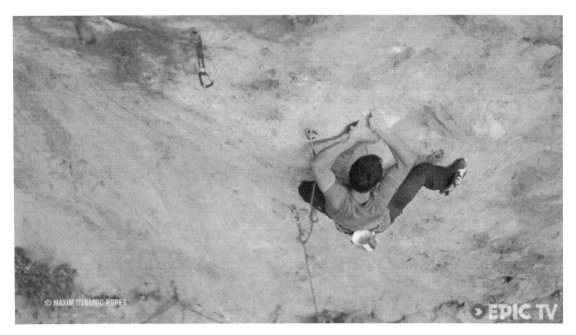

Type of Climbing

- Boulder
- Top Rope
- Free Solo
- Sport
- Trad
- Aid
- Big Wall

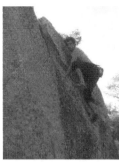 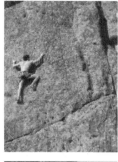 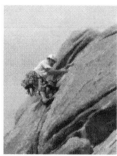
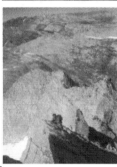 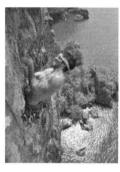 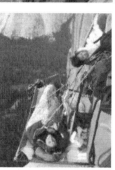

Copyright © 2019 Dr. Jared Vagy DPT

Publications

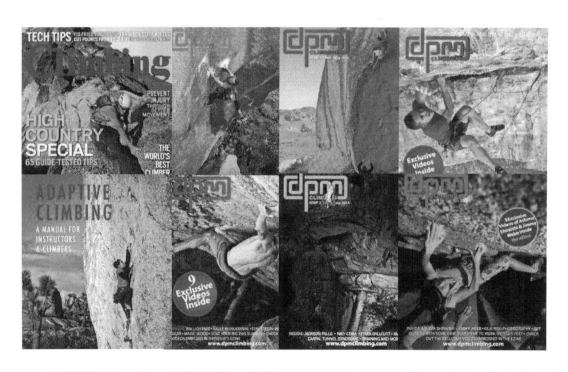

Books

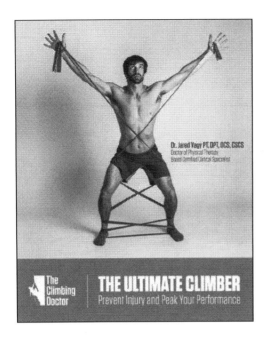
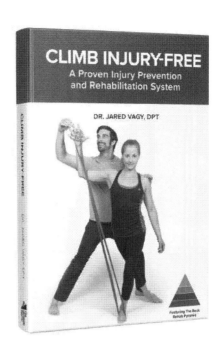

5 Advanced Concepts

1. **Mirroring Movement** (Climbing)
2. **Video Analysis** (Baseball)
3. **Dysfunctional Position** (Swimming)
4. **Kinetic Chain** (Tennis)
5. **Critical Events** (Volleyball)

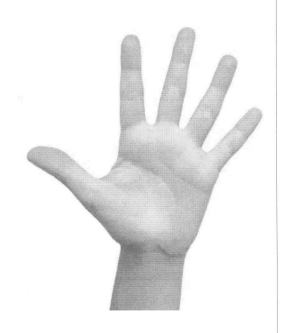

Copyright © 2017 Dr. Jared Vagy DPT

Mirror standing assessment

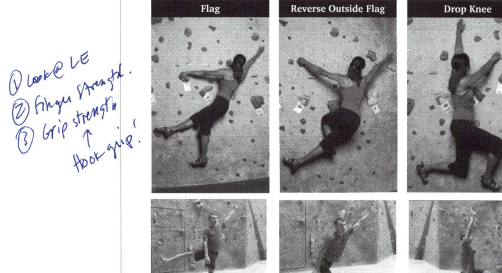

① look @ LE
② finger strength
③ Grip strength ↑ Hook grip!

Copyright © 2019 Dr. Jared Vagy DPT

Drop Knee

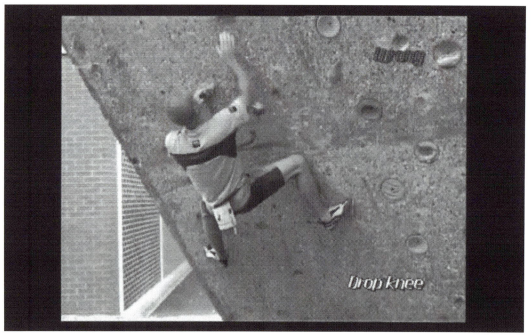

Copyright © 2019 Dr. Jared Vagy DPT

High Step

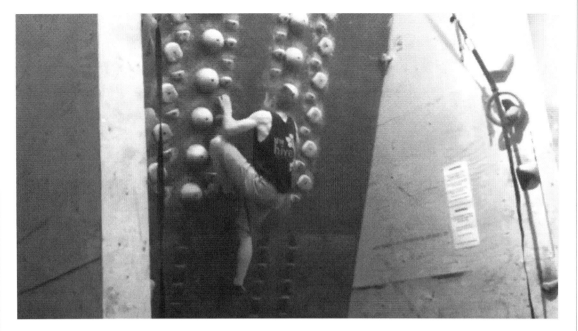

Flag and Reverse Outside Flag

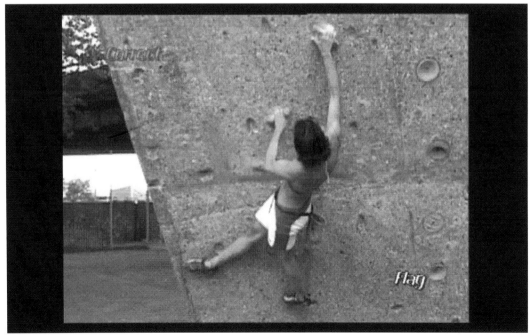

The Athlete Movement System: Upper Quarter

Neck Strain

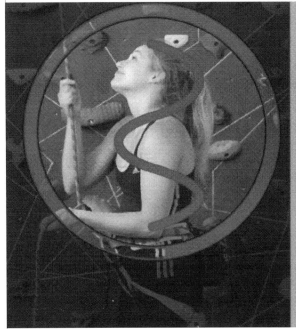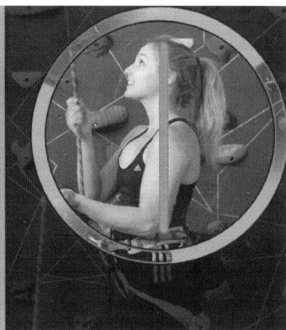

Copyright © 2019 Dr. Jared Vagy DPT

Shoulder Impingement

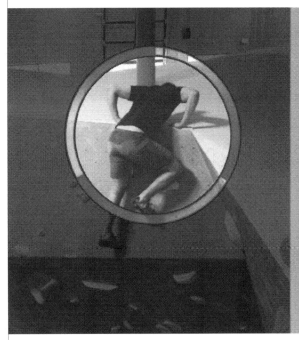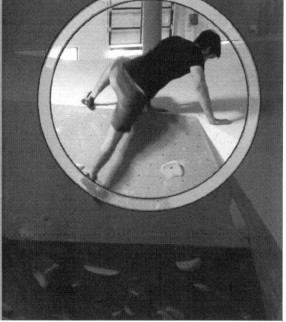

Copyright © 2019 Dr. Jared Vagy DPT

Medial Epicondylosis Video

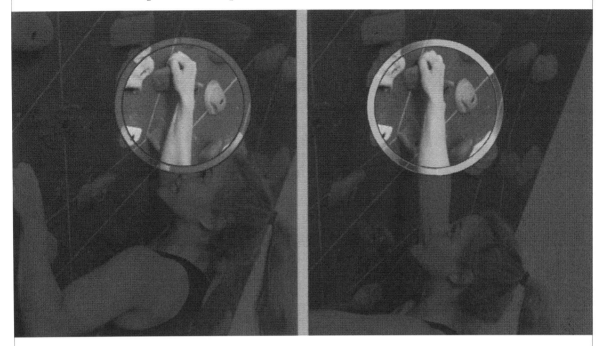

Baseball

Baseball

- Ancient Roots
  - 14th century France, contains an illustration of clerics.
  - Game's most direct antecedents are the English games of stoolball and "tut-ball."
  - 1830s a variety of bat-and-ball games recognizable as early forms of baseball in North America.

- Modern sport and recreation
  - 17.56 million in the United States have played in the past 12 months.

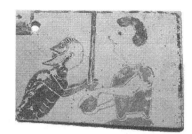

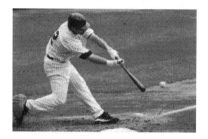

Throwing

The throwing motion facilitates the synchronization of the kinetic chain.
- The scapula plays a key role in the positioning of the glenoid, allowing for the necessary extremes of motion to occur without impingement. (Dillman 1993, Myers 2005)
- The greatest angular velocities and the largest change in rotation occur during the acceleration phase. (Pappas 1985)

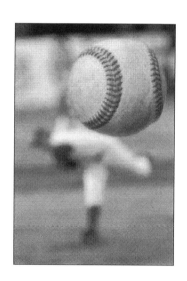

Throwing Critical Events

- ✓ Wind Up Phase
- ✓ Stride Phase
- ✓ Cocking Phase
  - ✓ Early Cocking
  - ✓ Late Cocking
- ✓ Acceleration Phase
- ✓ Deceleration Phase
- ✓ Follow Through Phase

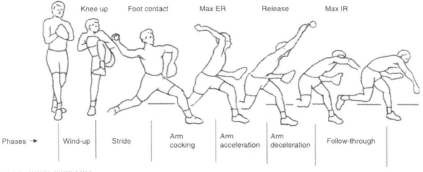

Copyright © 2019 Dr. Jared Vagy DPT

Motion Analysis of the Throw

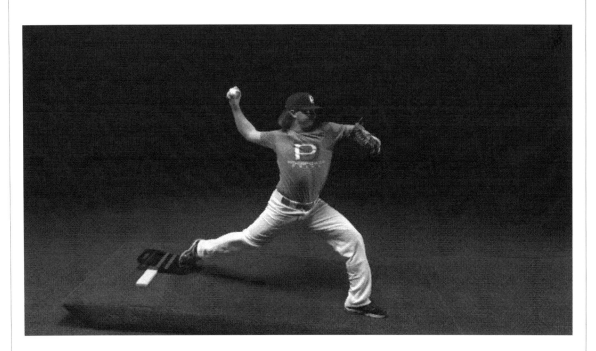

Copyright © 2019 Dr. Jared Vagy DPT

Problem

Current pitching assessment tool in literature is a 24-point checklist

- Not intended to identify pitchers with higher risk of injury
- Does not predict loads placed on the joint, pitchers' risk of injury, or performance
- Poor visual accuracy compared to motion capture

Phase	Variable
Foot contact	Preparatory movements
	Balance
	Hand separation
	Stride hip path
Stride	Stride length
	Stride offset
	Foot angle
	Knee flexion
	Horizontal adduction
	Abduction
	External rotation
	Elbow flexion
Arm cocking	Hip/shoulder rotation
	Trunk arching
	Use of glove arm
	Maximum elbow flexion
	Maximum external rotation
Ball Release	Trunk flexion
	Lateral trunk tilt
	Knee flexion
	Horizontal adduction
	Abduction
	Elbow flexion
Follow-through	Trunk flexion

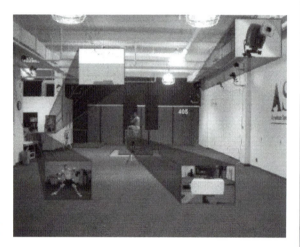

Copyright © 2019 Dr. Jared Vagy DPT

Solution

A targeted 6 point assessment tool linked to biomechanics stresses

Wind up -> Early Cocking	Forearm supination	Increases elbow vagus load and can lead to excessive shoulder horizontal abduction
Early Cocking -> Late Cocking	Open/closed foot position	Increases anterior forces at the shoulder
	Backward lean at stride foot contact	Increases shoulder and elbow joint loading
	Open shoulder	Increases horizontal abduction and stress on the anterior shoulder
	Decreased trunk to elbow angle at stride foot contact	Increases shoulder horizontal abduction. The scapula is placed in an unstable position if the humerus does not reach max height 93°+11°
Late Cocking -> Acceleration	Contralateral trunk lean at maximal shoulder external rotation	Increases proximal forces on the shoulder

Copyright © 2019 Dr. Jared Vagy DPT

Validated Pitching Error Scoring System

- 34 male pitchers 12-17 years old.
- Established intra and inter-rater reliability of previously studied biomechanical errors linked to elbow and shoulder injury.
- All 6 errors tested had acceptable intra-rater reliability.
- 3 out of 6 biomechanical errors had acceptable inter-rater reliability
    - Stride foot position at stride foot contact
    - Backward lean at stride foot contact
    - Contralateral lean at max humeral lateral rotation

Established the reliability of previously studied biomechanical errors to create a valid and reliable assessment tool to identify faulty pitching mechanics, which predispose these athletes to serious upper extremity injuries.

Quatromoni, Emily. Reliability of a visual observation pitching assessment in adolescent pitchers. Diss. The University of North Carolina at Chapel Hill, 2015.

Motion Analysis of the Throw

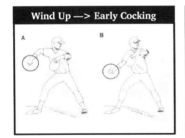
Wind Up —> Early Cocking

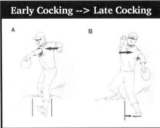
Early Cocking --> Late Cocking

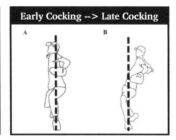
Early Cocking --> Late Cocking

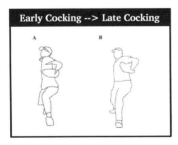
Early Cocking --> Late Cocking

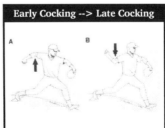
Early Cocking --> Late Cocking

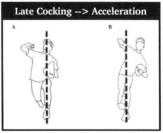
Late Cocking --> Acceleration

↑ lean = ↑ speed =↑
Oyama et al. AJSM 2013.

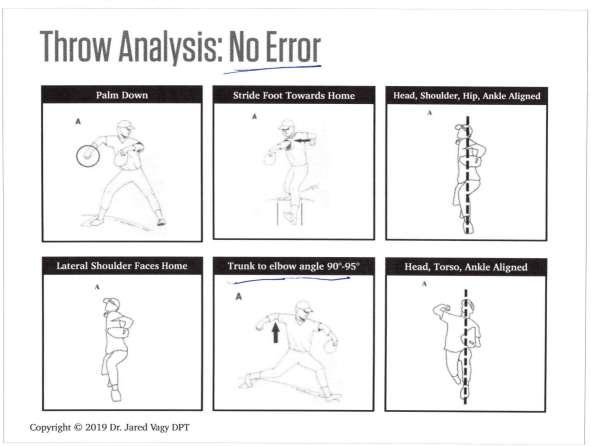

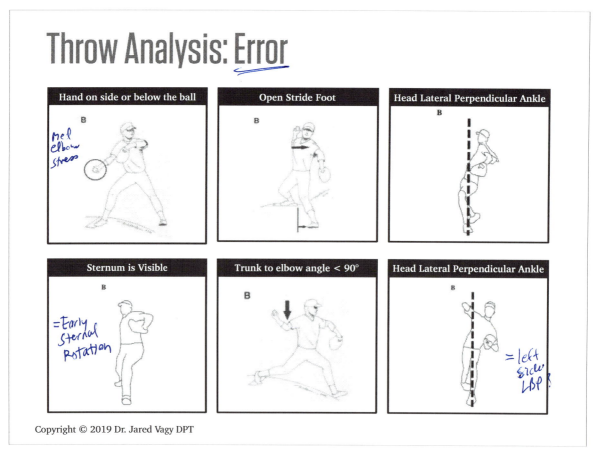

Motion Analysis of the Throw

| Stride Foot to Home | Head, Shoulder, Hip, Ankle Aligned | Palm Down |
| Lateral Shoulder Face Home | Head, Torso, Ankle Aligned | Trunk to elbow angle 90°-95° |

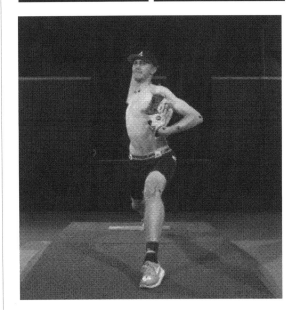
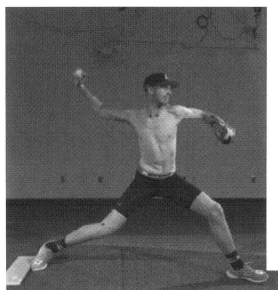

Little League Elbow

- Excessive repetitive stress to growth plate at the elbow.
- Imbalance between growth of long bone and length of muscles/tendons.
- Age 9-14
- Curveballs and sliders increase risk:
  - Curveballs = 1.6x more likely to have arm pain (Yang 2014)
  - Sliders = 86% more likely to have elbow pain (Lyman 2002)

Prevention: Regulate and monitor pitch counts and take into account skeletal maturity.

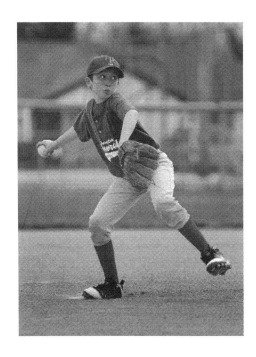

Copyright © 2019 Dr. Jared Vagy DPT

UCL Sprain

One of the primary stabilizers of the elbow joint:
- The UCL is usually sprained in position of elbow flexion when elbow has decreased osseous stability.

From late cocking phase to release:
- .03 seconds time
- 7000 degrees per second
- Rate of 20 arm rotations per second

Prevention: Regulate and monitor pitch counts and awareness of self arm care.

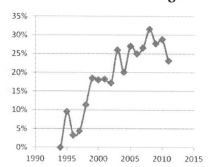

UCL Reconstructive Surgeries

Total number of surgeries at Andrews Sports Med clinic

| Position of elbow flexion |
| Elbow destabilized |
| High pitching speed |
| Ligamentous stress |

Copyright © 2019 Dr. Jared Vagy DPT

5 Advanced Concepts

1. **Mirroring Movement** (Climbing)
2. **Video Analysis** (Baseball)
3. **Dysfunctional Position** (Swimming)
4. **Kinetic Chain** (Tennis)
5. **Critical Events** (Volleyball)

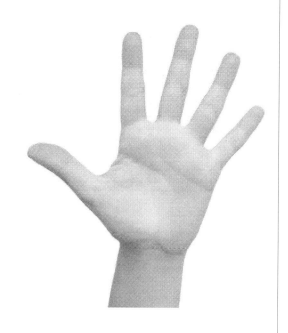

Copyright © 2017 Dr. Jared Vagy DPT

Movement Analysis with Technology

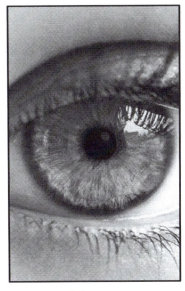

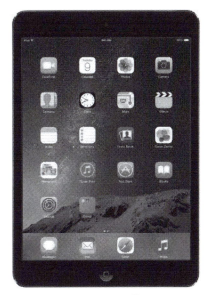

Eye Or Eye Pad

Technology makes it simple to catch movements difficult to see with the naked eye

Technology and Apps

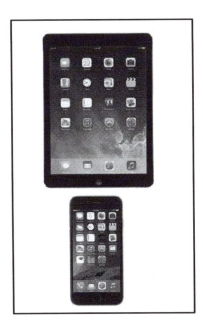

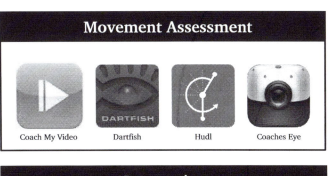

Movement Assessment: Coach My Video, Dartfish, Hudl, Coaches Eye

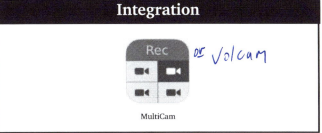

Integration: MultiCam — or Volcam

Technology and Apps

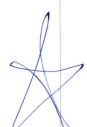

MultiCam
Rec

- Adequate lighting
- Sunlight direction
- At least 240 frames per second
- Limit frontal plane variation

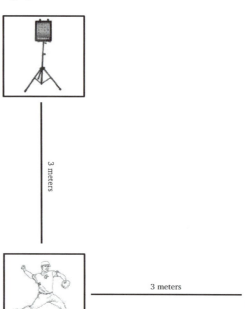

3 meters

3 meters

Motion Analysis of Throw

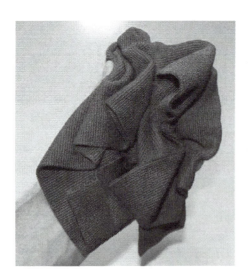

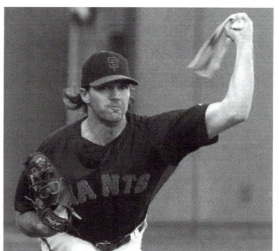

Swimming

Swimming

- Ancient roots
  - 2,000 B.C is the first record of swimming.
  - Paintings of swimming date back to over 10,000 years ago.
  - 1828 first indoor swimming pool in England.
  - 1896 Olympic sport in the first modern games.

- Modern sport and recreation
  - 76 million swimmers in the United States.
  - A fast growing modern sport.

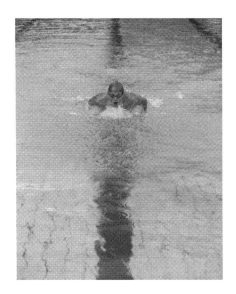

Common Strokes

- Freestyle
- Breaststroke
- Butterfly
- Backstroke

Most Common Injury Diagnosis

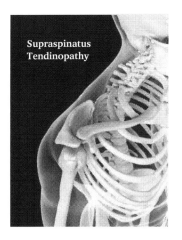

Most common diagnosis *(Sein et al. 2008)*

- Supraspinatus tendinopathy is the most common cause of pain in the swimmer's shoulder.
- 69% of elite swimmers
- Increased swim time and weekly distance correlated significantly with supraspinatus tendinopathy.

High Incidence of Shoulder Pain

Shoulder pain by category (McMaster 1993)

- 47% of 10 to 18-year-old swimmers

- 66% of senior swimmers

- 73% of elite swimmers

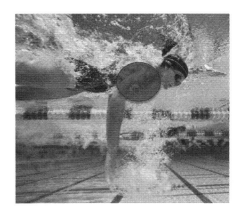

Shoulder pain overall (McMaster 1993)

- 47-73% of competitive swimmers reported shoulder pain (McMaster 1993)

Copyright © 2019 Dr. Jared Vagy DPT

High Volume of Shoulder Rotations

- The average competitive swimmer swims approximately 60,000 to 80,000 meters per week.

- Approximately 8-10 strokes per 25-meter lap

- Each shoulder performs 30,000 rotations each week

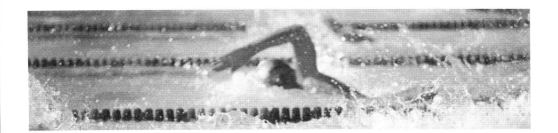

Copyright © 2019 Dr. Jared Vagy DPT

Gender Differences

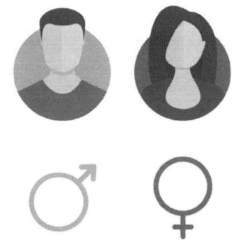

- **Higher ratio of female** compared to male presentations with shoulder pain. *(Bot et al 2005)*

A Reason for Gender Difference (McMaster et al. 1998)

- Significant correlation between shoulder laxity and shoulder pain in swimmers.

- One reason why women may be more susceptible to shoulder pain is from increased hormonal laxity.

- Be aware of overtraining during menstrual cycle.

Other Common Injury Diagnoses

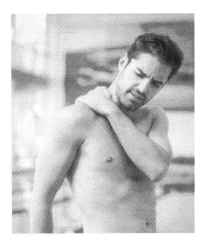

Other Common Diagnoses

- Facet dysfunction and neck strain
- High percentage of all swimmers
- Poor neck rotation mechanics, breathing one side repetitively, and increased frequency of rotation and extension during stroke.

Copyright © 2019 Dr. Jared Vagy DPT

Biomechanics of the Swim Stroke

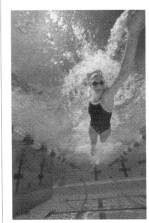 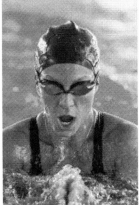 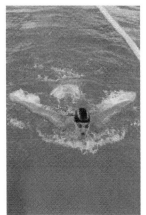 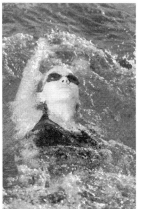

Freestyle

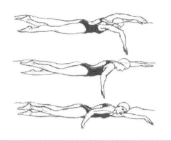 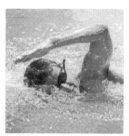

The shoulder joint is particularly vulnerable with 92% of propulsive forces coming from the upper extremity.

Mean duration of impingement position was 24.8%. (Yanai et al. 2000)
  14.4% during pulling
  10.4% during recovery

Freestyle is the fastest of the 4 strokes and has the most research.

Freestyle Video

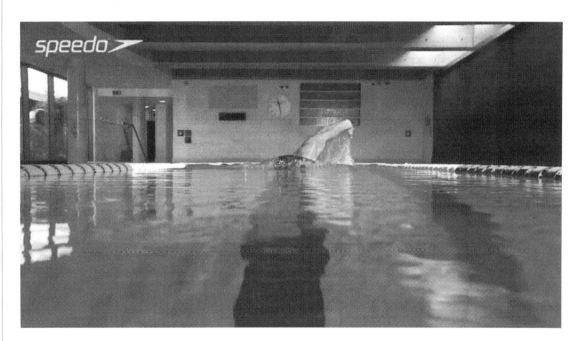

Freestyle Critical Events

✓ Pull-Through Phase = hand in water
  ✓ Early — Finger enters the water -> Max elbow extension
  ✓ Mid — Max elbow extension -> Hand crosses the chest
  ✓ Late — Hand crosses the chest -> Little finger exit the water

✓ Recovery Phase = hand out of water
  ✓ Early — Finger exits water -> Humeral abd and lateral rot
  ✓ Late — Humeral abd and lateral rot -> Arm is in position for hand entry

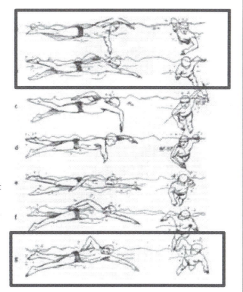

Copyright © 2019 Dr. Jared Vagy DPT

Muscle Actions

squeeze shoulder blades

Early Recovery
- Posterior Deltoid
- Middle Deltoid
- Rhomboids

Mid-Recovery
- Middle Deltoid
- Upper Trapezius
- Serratus Anterior
- Infraspinatus

Late Recovery
- Middle Deltoid
- Anterior Deltoid
- Serratus Anterior
- Rhomboids
- Subscapularis

End of Pulling
- Subscapularis
- Posterior/Middle Deltoids
- Supraspinatus

Glide/Reach
- Anterior/Middle Deltoid
- Upper Trapezius
- Rhomboids

Rely on SA for scap control

Late Pull Through
- Latissimus Dorsi
- Subscapularis

Mid Pull Through
- Serratus Anterior
- Pectoralis Major
- Latissimus Dorsi

Early Pull Through
- Pectoralis Major
- Teres Minor (extension)

Copyright © 2019 Dr. Jared Vagy DPT

Research: Shoulder Pain & EMG

- Swimmers with and without shoulder pain were asked to complete an upper extremity task.
- 17 elite swimmers with shoulder pain were compared to matched control elite swimmers without shoulder pain
- EMG activity of upper trapezius, anterior scalene, and sternocleidomastoid were monitored during a seated functional task.

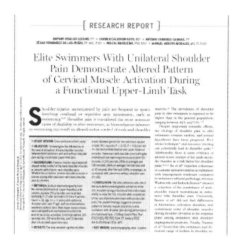

Subjects with shoulder pain had greater upper trapezius, sternocleidomastoid and scalene EMG

Higdalgo-Lozano A, Calderon-Soto C, Domingo-Camara A, et al. Elite Swimmers with Unilateral Shoulder Pain Demonstrate Altered Pattern of Cervical Muscle Activation During a Functional Upper Limb Task. J Orthop Sports PT, 2012. 42(6) 552-558

Poor Shoulder Mechanics (Scovazzo et al. 1991)

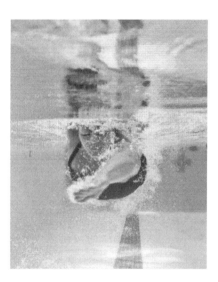

Pull-through Phase
- Arm closer to midline
- Decreased upward rotation
- Decreased serratus anterior activity
- Increased rhomboids activity

Recovery Phase
- Early hand exit

Copyright © 2019 Dr. Jared Vagy DPT

Poor Neck Mechanics

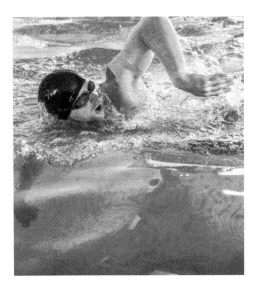

- Rotating the head off axis
- Rotating neck too much
- Looking too far forward
- Breathing only on one side

Backstroke

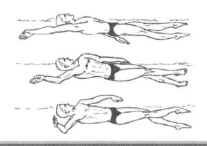
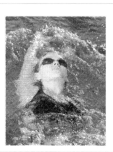

- Can be a good training alternative because muscle actions are opposite the force of gravity

- Easier to breathe

Backstroke Video

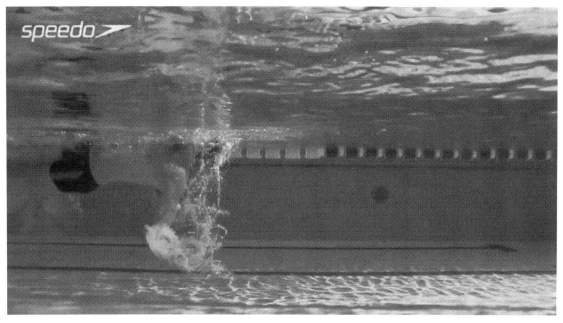

Backstroke Critical Events

Pull-through Phase

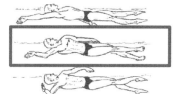

Recovery Phase

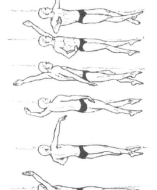

Poor Shoulder and Neck Mechanics

Shoulder
- Not rotating the trunk to clear the shoulder

Neck
- Excessive cervical extension

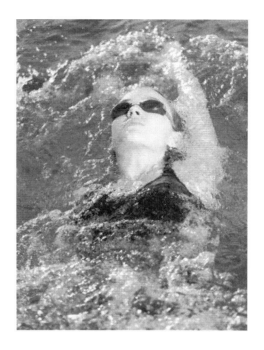

Copyright © 2019 Dr. Jared Vagy DPT

Butterfly

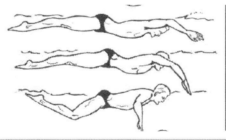
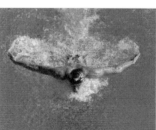

- Similar sequence to the freestyle but the arms are used synchronously

- Different from freestyle because there is not thoracic rotation, only thoracic extension

- Uses the hips to generate power

Butterfly Video

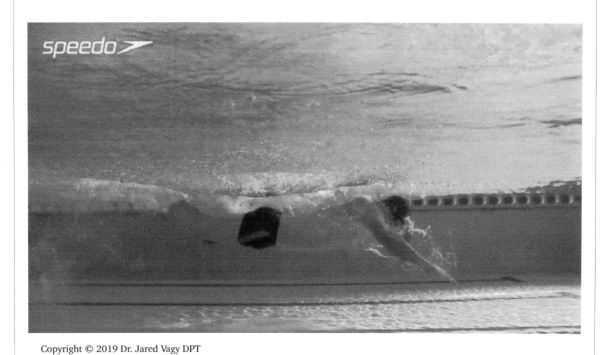

Butterfly Critical Events

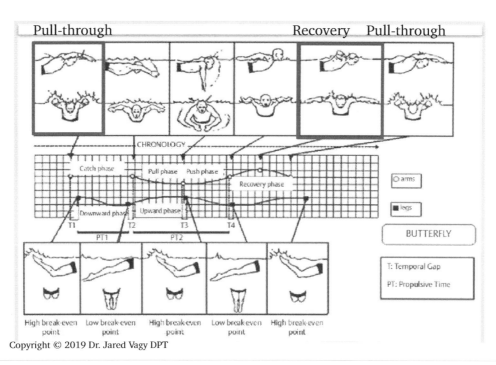

Butterfly Critical Events

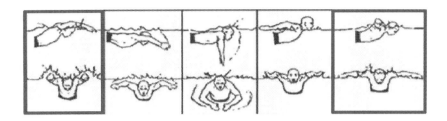

- ✓ Pull-Through Phase
  - ✓ Early
  - ✓ Mid
  - ✓ Late
- ✓ Recovery Phase
  - ✓ Early
  - ✓ Late

Copyright © 2019 Dr. Jared Vagy DPT

Freestyle and Butterfly are Similar

Freestyle

Butterfly

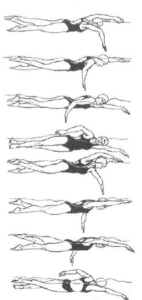
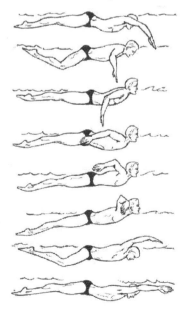

Copyright © 2019 Dr. Jared Vagy DPT

Poor Shoulder Mechanics (Pink et al. 1993)

Pull-through phase
- Narrow hand entry
- Decreased serratus anterior muscle activity

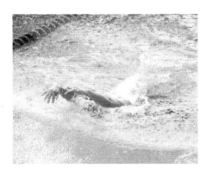 VS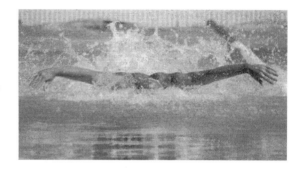

Poor Neck Mechanics

- Weak kick
- Lack of upper body strength
- Poor timing by breathing too late

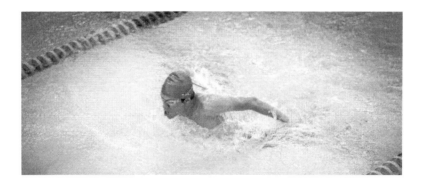

Breaststroke

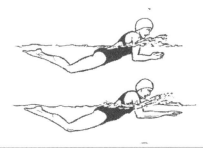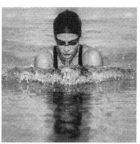

Upper Body Similar to Butterfly
- The arm motion in the breaststroke initially resembles the beginning pull of a butterfly stroke.

Upper Body Different from Butterfly
- Does not continue with the forearms passing under the body to the level of the hips.

Breaststroke Video

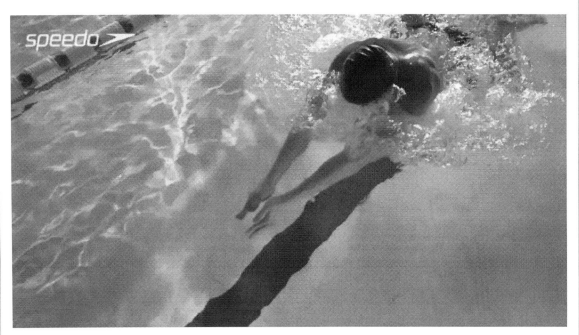

Breaststroke Critical Events

Glide

Pull-through

Reach

Glide

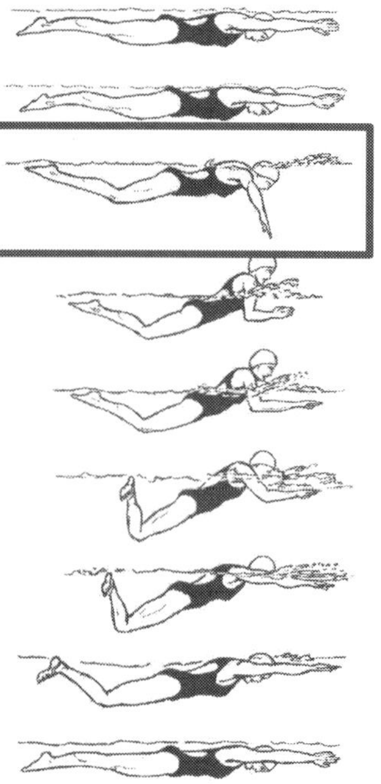

Freestyle and Breaststroke Differences

Freestyle   Breaststroke

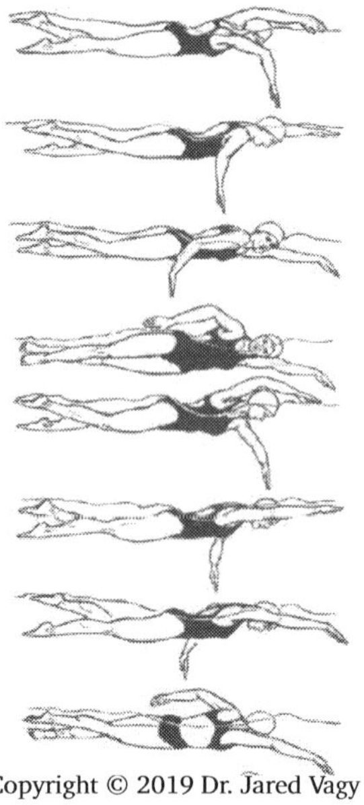

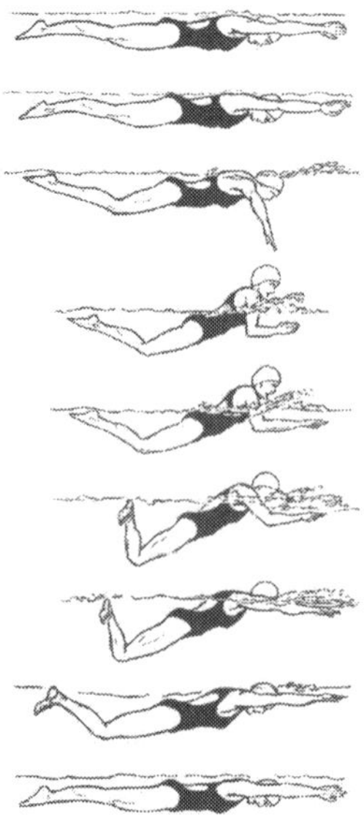

- Breaststroke has a longer recovery phase
- Freestyle has a much longer pulling phase

Poor Shoulder and Neck Mechanics (Scovazzo et al. 1991)

Shoulder
- During pull-through, swimmers with painful shoulders had increased Latissimus Dorsi, Upper Trapezius and Subscapularis activity.

Neck
- Tilting head back to breathe.

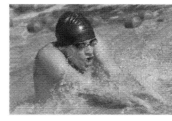

5 Advanced Concepts

1. **Mirroring Movement** (Climbing)
2. **Video Analysis** (Baseball)
3. **Dysfunctional Position** (Swimming)
4. **Kinetic Chain** (Tennis)
5. **Critical Events** (Volleyball)

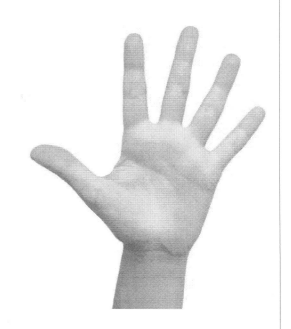

Apply The Movement System

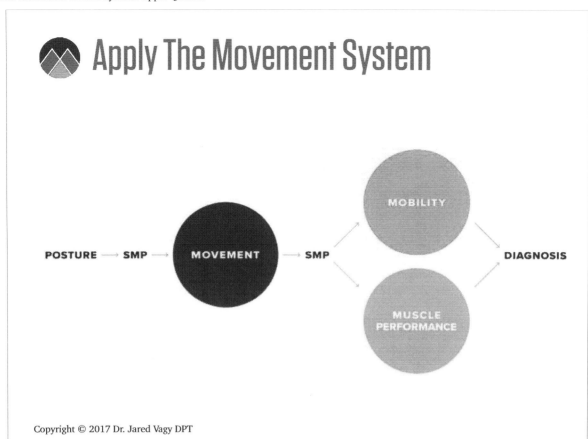

Assess the Dysfunctional Position

What happens to the technique when the demand increases?

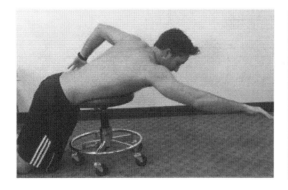
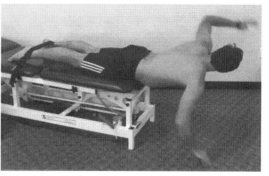

Assess the Dysfunctional Position

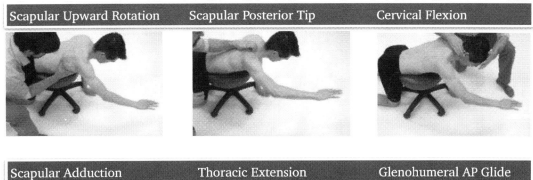

Tennis

Tennis

- Ancient Roots
  - 12th century northern France, where a ball was struck with the palm of the hand.
  - 16th century is when racquets came into use.
  - 19th century the modern game originated in England .

- Modern sport and recreation
  - Tennis is played by millions of recreational players and is also a popular worldwide spectator sport.
  - 200 countries affiliated with the International Tennis Federation.

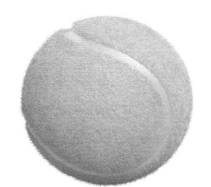

Common Strokes

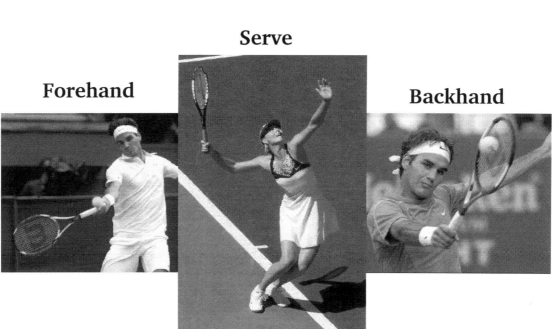

Forehand — Serve — Backhand

w/ Backhand (Single hand)
Novice – 13° flexion (wrist) w/ ↑ flexion
Pro – ~30° extension w/ ↑ extension (wrist)

Tennis Elbow

De Smedt et al. 2007

Lateral epicondylitis

- Tendinopathy of wrist extensors
- One of most common overuse injuries in tennis
- More common in the recreational player

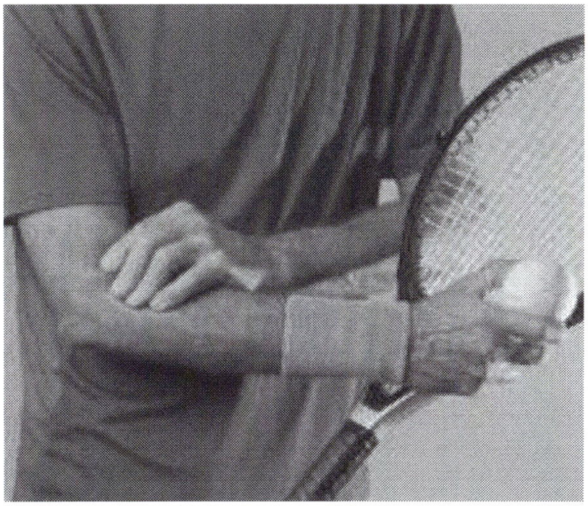

Incidence

- 35% to 51% – Mostly recreational players.

High Training Volume

Increased training time weekly may lead to increased pain

(Kitai et al. 1986)

- Players with lateral epicondylitis:
  - 8 hours per week
- Pain free players
  - 5.5 hours per week

Increased training hours may lead to increased pain

(Gruchow et al. 1979)

- Players with lateral epicondylitis
  - 2 hours per day
- Pain free players
  - less than 2 hours per day

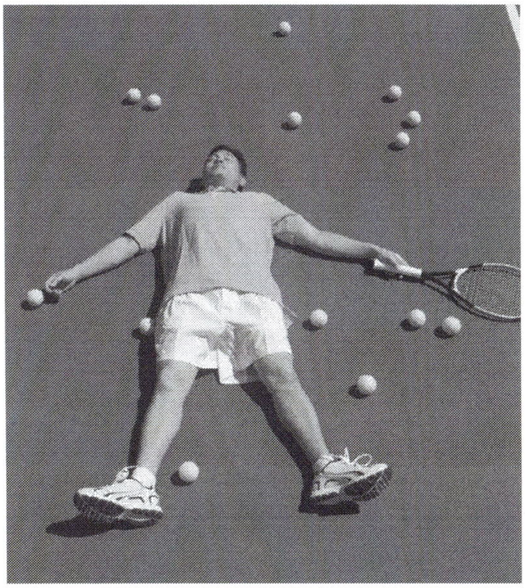

Bigger Head Equals Less Pain
Hennig et al. 1992

Reduced arm vibration with increased racket head size

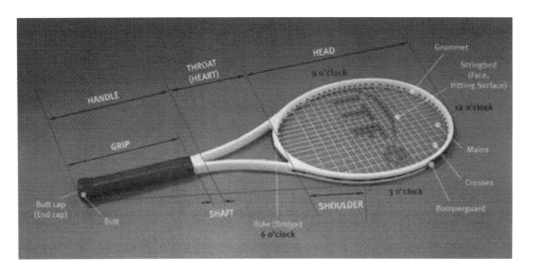

Wrist Pain
Smedt et al. 2007

Common Diagnoses
- Extensor Carpi Ulnaris tendonitis
- Triangular Fibrocartilage Complex pathology
- Flexor Carpi Radialis tendonitis
- DeQuervian's tendinopathy
- Intersection syndrome

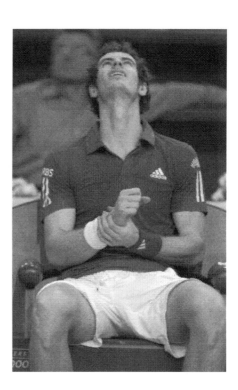

Different Grips = Different Pain

Grips
- Continental
- Eastern
- Semiwestern
- Full western

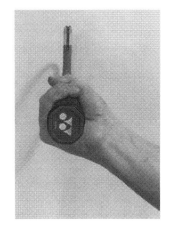
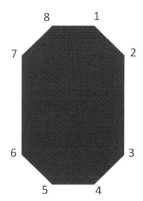

Injuries from Tennis Forehand

Ulnar-sided injuries more common with Western or Semiwestern grips
- Extensor Carpi Ulnaris tendonitis
- Triangular Fibrocartilage Complex pathology

Radial-sided injuries more common in players with the eastern grip
- Flexor Carpi Radialis tendonitis
- DeQuervian's tendinopathy
- Intersection syndrome

Western
Index Knuckle on bevel 5
Hypothenar on Bevel 5

Semiwestern
Index Knuckle on Bevel 4
Hypothenar on Bevel 4

Eastern
Index Knuckle on Bevel 3
Hypothenar on Bevel 3

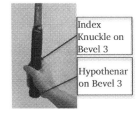

Volleyball

Tennis Serve Biomechanics

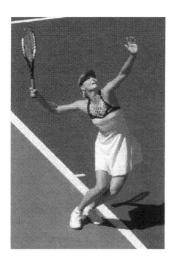
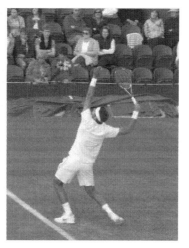
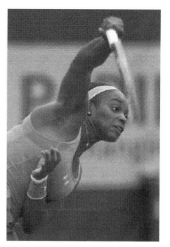

High Incidence of Shoulder Pain _{Kibler 2000}

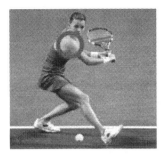
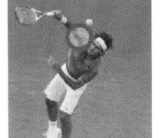

- 25 to 47% of all arm injuries are shoulder injuries
- 7 to 16% of all reported injuries are shoulder injuries

- **High loads**
    - Serve: arm velocity 72 mph
    - One-hand backhand: arm velocity 34 mph
    - Open stance forehand: 46 mph

- Shoulder should only produce 13% of total kinetic energy for entire service motion (Lintner

Copyright © 2019 Dr. Jared Vagy DPT

The Tennis Serve

- 60% of all strokes
- Goal:
    - Optimal ball speed
    - Efficient force production
    - Max torque for minimal force
    - Minimize joint loading
    - Minimize degrees of freedom
- Types of Serves
    - Flat
    - Slice
    - Topspin/Kick

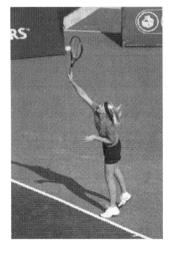
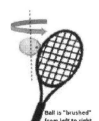
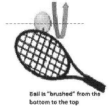
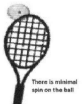

Ball is "brushed" from left to right | Ball is "brushed" from the bottom to the top | There is minimal spin on the ball

Copyright © 2019 Dr. Jared Vagy DPT

Serve Video

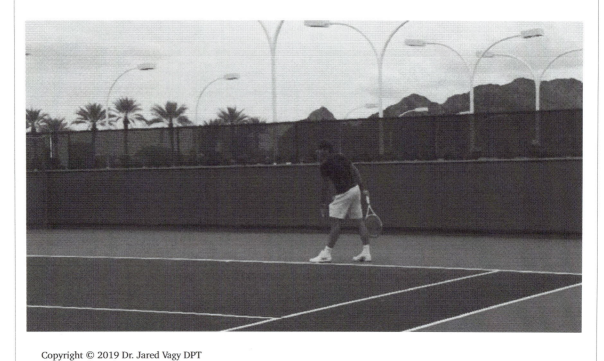

Service Motion

Max Sh. Stressors
↓   ↓

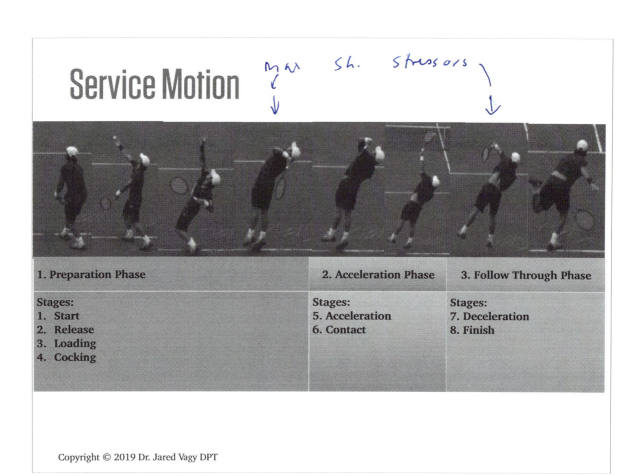

1. Preparation Phase	2. Acceleration Phase	3. Follow Through Phase
Stages: 1. Start 2. Release 3. Loading 4. Cocking	Stages: 5. Acceleration 6. Contact	Stages: 7. Deceleration 8. Finish

The Kinetic Chain and The Serve

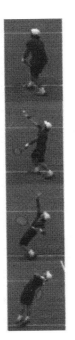

Phase	Stage	Critical Events
1. Preparation	1. Start	
	2. Release	From start to when ball is released
	3. Loading	From ball release to position of max knee flexion and elbow's lowest vertical position
	4. Cocking	From maximum knee flexion to maximum (shoulder external rotation.) Tip of racket pointing to ground

Copyright © 2019 Dr. Jared Vagy DPT

The Kinetic Chain and The Serve

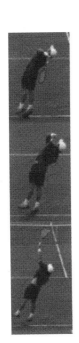

Phase	Stage	Critical Events
2. Acceleration	5. Acceleration	From end of cocking to contact
	6. Contact	Near Instantaneous impact of ball and racket

Copyright © 2019 Dr. Jared Vagy DPT

The Athlete Movement System: Upper Quarter

The Kinetic Chain and The Serve

Phase	Stage	Critical Events
3. Follow Through	7. Deceleration	After contact until end of slowing down of upper and lower body movement
	8. Finish	Point of stability at end of serve prior to next stroke

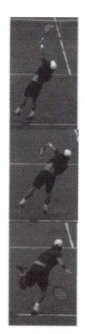

MVIC
RTC : 30-35%
SA : 53%

Copyright © 2019 Dr. Jared Vagy DPT

Critical Events of the Tennis Serve: Loading

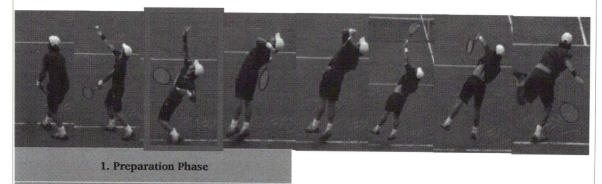

1. Preparation Phase

Stages:
1. Start
2. Release
3. Loading
4. Cocking

- 6 Critical Events in Loading Stage

*Based on Observational Tennis Serve Analysis Tool
Myers et al 2017

Copyright © 2019 Dr. Jared Vagy DPT

Phase 1: Stage 3 Loading

- 6 Important critical events that distinguish high vs low ranked players

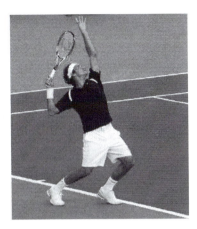

1. Knee position
2. Back Hip Counter Rotation
3. Posterior Hip Tilt and Loading
4. X-angle
5. Trunk Rotation
6. Arm Position

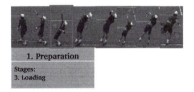

1. Preparation
Stages:
3. Loading

Critical Event #1: Knee Loading

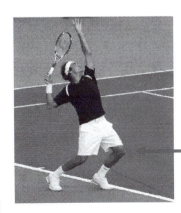

Normal Mechanics	Non-Optimal Mechanics	Result
Knee Flexion >15 degrees	Knee Flexion < 15 degrees	• Increased load on anterior shoulder and medial elbow. • 23 to 27% increased loads in horizontal adduction and rotation at the shoulder and valgus load at elbow

The Athlete Movement System: Upper Quarter

Critical Event #2: Back Hip Counter Rotation

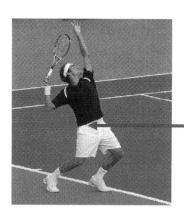

Normal	Non-Optimal	Result
Back hip is rotating away from the net	Back hip is not rotating away from the net	• Increased load on shoulder and trunk. • Difficulty with energy transfer through trunk

Copyright © 2019 Dr. Jared Vagy DPT

Critical Event #3: Posterior Hip Tilt and Load

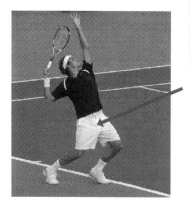

Normal	Non-Optimal	Result
Posterior hip is dropping to the ground and back leg is loaded	No tilt of hips. No pressure on back leg.	• Increased load on shoulder and trunk. • Difficulty with energy transfer through trunk

Copyright © 2019 Dr. Jared Vagy DPT

Critical Event #4: X-angle

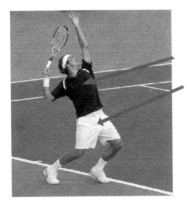

Normal Mechanics	Non-Optimal Mechanics	Result
X-angle (shoulders rotating past hips) approximately 30 deg. with controlled lordosis	• Hyperlordosis • X-angle > 30 degrees (shoulders too far behind the hips) • X-angle <30 degrees (shoulders do not rotate enough past hips)	• Increased load on shoulder and trunk. • Difficulty with energy transfer through trunk

Critical Event #5: Trunk Rotation

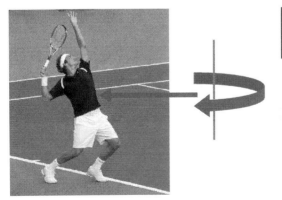

Normal Mechanics	Non-Optimal Mechanics	Result
Trunk Rotation around a vertical axis	No trunk rotation. Only lateral bend or extension through spine.	Difficulty with energy transfer through trunk

Critical Event #6: Arm Position

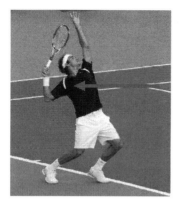

Normal Mechanics	Non-Optimal Mechanics	Result
Shoulder in line with the plane of the scapula	• Hypercocking: shoulder behind plane of scapula • Hypococking: shoulder in front of plane of scapula	Increased strain to rotator cuff and shoulder; anterior/posterior impingement

Non-Optimal Mechanics: What Are They?

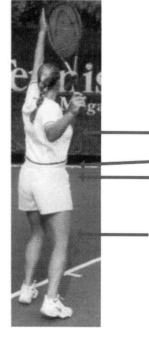

- No Backwards Trunk Rotation; X angle = 0 deg
- Inadequate Hip Tilt
- Inadequate Hip Rotation
- Knee Flexion Angle < 15 deg

The Athlete Movement System: Upper Quarter

Critical Events of the Tennis Serve: Contact

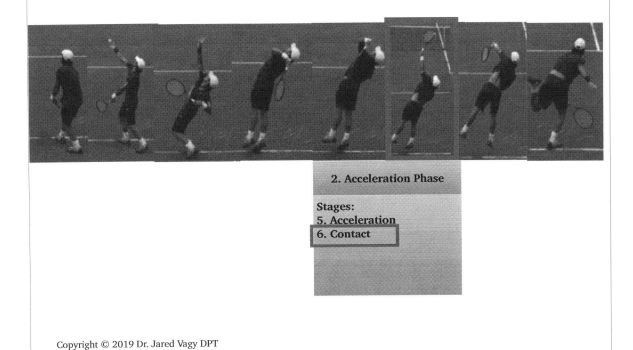

2. Acceleration Phase

Stages:
5. Acceleration
6. Contact

Copyright © 2019 Dr. Jared Vagy DPT

Critical Events of the Tennis Serve: Contact

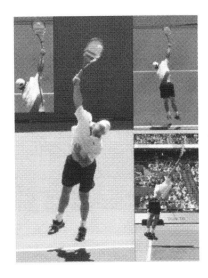

Joint Range	Optimal Positioning at ball contact
Shoulder Abduction	110 deg +/- 15 deg abduction
Trunk Flexion	48 deg +/-7 deg from horizontal
Elbow flexion	20 deg +/-4 deg
Front Knee Flexion	24 deg +/- 14 deg
Wrist Extension	15 deg +/-8 deg

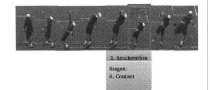

2. Acceleration

Stages:
6. Contact

Copyright © 2019 Dr. Jared Vagy DPT

Critical Events: Loading to Contact

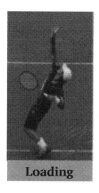 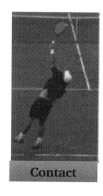

Loading   Contact

- High trunk muscle activation between Stage 3 and 6
- Power generation through trunk
  - Reversal of the X-angle
    - 20% reduction in kinetic energy from trunk requires 34% more velocity OR 70% increase in mass to achieve same kinetic energy to hand
    - Leads to increase strain on shoulder and arm

Copyright © 2019 Dr. Jared Vagy DPT

---

5 Advanced Concepts

1. **Mirroring Movement** (Climbing)
2. **Video Analysis** (Baseball)
3. **Dysfunctional Position** (Swimming)
4. **Kinetic Chain** (Tennis)
5. **Critical Events** (Volleyball)

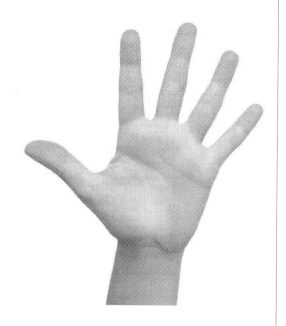

Copyright © 2017 Dr. Jared Vagy DPT

Utilize the Kinetic Chain

use velocity app for modified version of this.

- Assessment of Trunk Rotational Power
- Field Test of Cowley and Swenson
- Power = (Force X Distance) / time
  - Force: weight of medicine ball (2.72 kg) in Newtons
  - Distance: meters
  - Time: seconds

	Good Serve Mechanics	Poor Serve Mechanics
Power	185.2 Watts	118.76 Watts

correlation 5

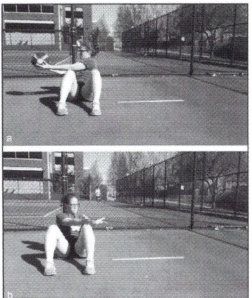

Myers et al 2017

Utilize the Kinetic Chain

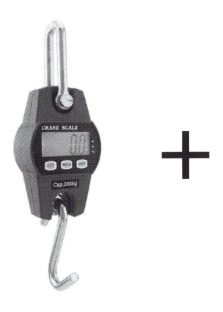 +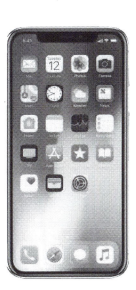

Volleyball

- Ancient Roots
  - The first rules, written down by William G Morgan 1895.
  - First played at the YMCA where Alfred Halstead noticed the volleying nature of the game called it volleyball.

- Modern sport and recreation
  - The third highest sport for female participation at the high school level
  - The greatest number of boys' teams are in Southern California.
  - For every boy currently competing in high school volleyball, more than eight girls are involved.

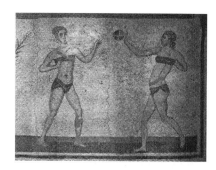

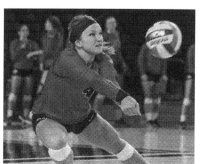

Volleyball Spike

- Of the overhead volleyball skills, the spike is perhaps the most explosive.
  (Reeser 2010)

- The majority of force imparted to the ball during a spike originates from the torso:
  - During a spike, the scapula is involved in transferring kinetic energy to the upper limb.
  - The scapula provides a stable base of support so that the upper limb can be correctly positioned in space during the performance of overhead skills.

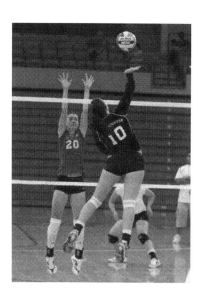

Volleyball Critical Events

✓ Wind Up Phase
✓ Cocking Phase
✓ Acceleration Phase
   ✓ Ball Contact
✓ Deceleration Phase
✓ Follow Through Phase

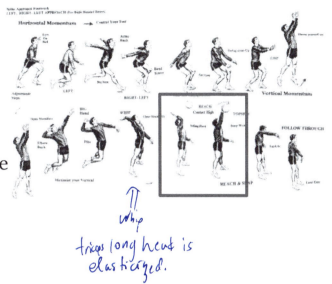

whip
triceps long head is elasticized.

Kinetic chain Thomas test
- add Sh flex. then elbow flexion

Volleyball Critical Events

Right hand spike
(L) → (R) → (L)
med long short
slow → fast
straight → 45°(R) → 90°(L) (leg position)
forward - back - up (arm position)

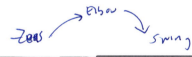
Zeus → Elbow → Swing

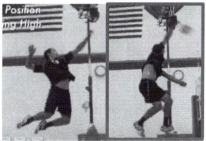

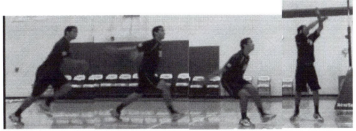

✓ Wind Up Phase
✓ Cocking Phase
✓ Acceleration Phase
   ✓ Ball Contact
✓ Deceleration Phase
✓ Follow Through Phase

The Athlete Movement System: Upper Quarter

Motion Analysis of the Spike

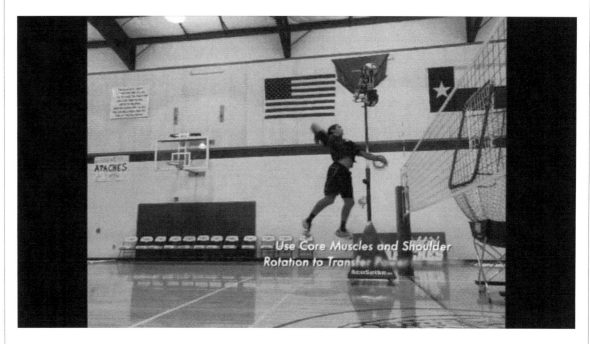

Use Core Muscles and Shoulder Rotation to Transfer...

Copyright © 2019 Dr. Jared Vagy DPT

5 Advanced Concepts

1. **Mirroring Movement** (Climbing)
2. **Video Analysis** (Baseball)
3. **Dysfunctional Position** (Swimming)
4. **Kinetic Chain** (Tennis)
5. **Critical Events** (Volleyball)

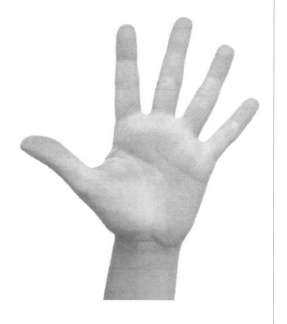

Copyright © 2017 Dr. Jared Vagy DPT

Motion Analysis of the Spike

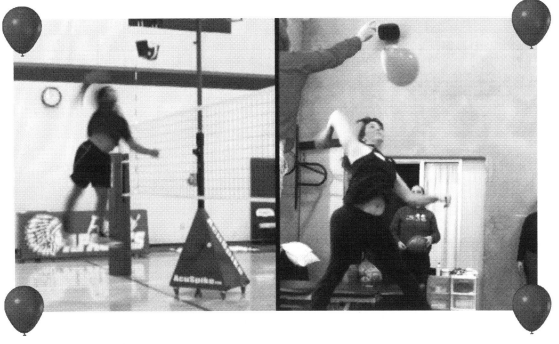

Day 1 Summary

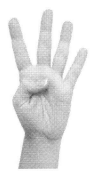
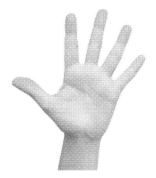

4 Foundational Concepts
- Movement Science Framework
- Relative Flexibility
- Joint Centration
- Muscle Performance

5 Advanced Concepts
- Mirroring Movement
- Video Analysis
- Dysfunctional Position
- Kinetic Chain
- Critical Events

The Treatment Pyramid

The Application of The Movement System into the Treatment of Sport Injury

Jared Vagy PT, DPT, OCS, CSCS

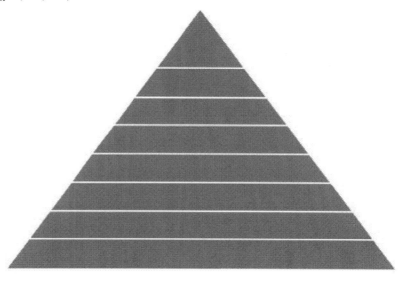

Copyright © 2019 Dr. Jared Vagy DPT

Course Schedule Day 2

- **8am-9am:** Lecture: The Treatment Pyramid Part 1
- **9am-12pm:** Lab: The Treatment Pyramid Part 1
- **12-1PM:** Lunch
- **1-2PM:** Lecture: The Treatment Pyramid Part 2
- **2-3PM:** Lab: The Treatment Pyramid Part 2
- **3-4PM:** Lab: Putting it All Together
- **4-4:30PM:** Lecture: Wrap up

Copyright © 2019 Dr. Jared Vagy DPT

Day 2 Objectives

- Learn the framework of a rehabilitation pyramid. Utilize the pyramid to sequence and organize your treatments.
- Utilize movement based treatment techniques of joint centration, post isometric relaxation, gravity induced inhibition and muscular facilitation.
- Use the 5 key resistance band concepts to develop exercises for athletes that target the entire movement system.
- Understand the relationship between neuromuscular chains and muscle slings and how to use their properties to enhance your treatments to progress into sport specific skill.

Treatment Pyramid

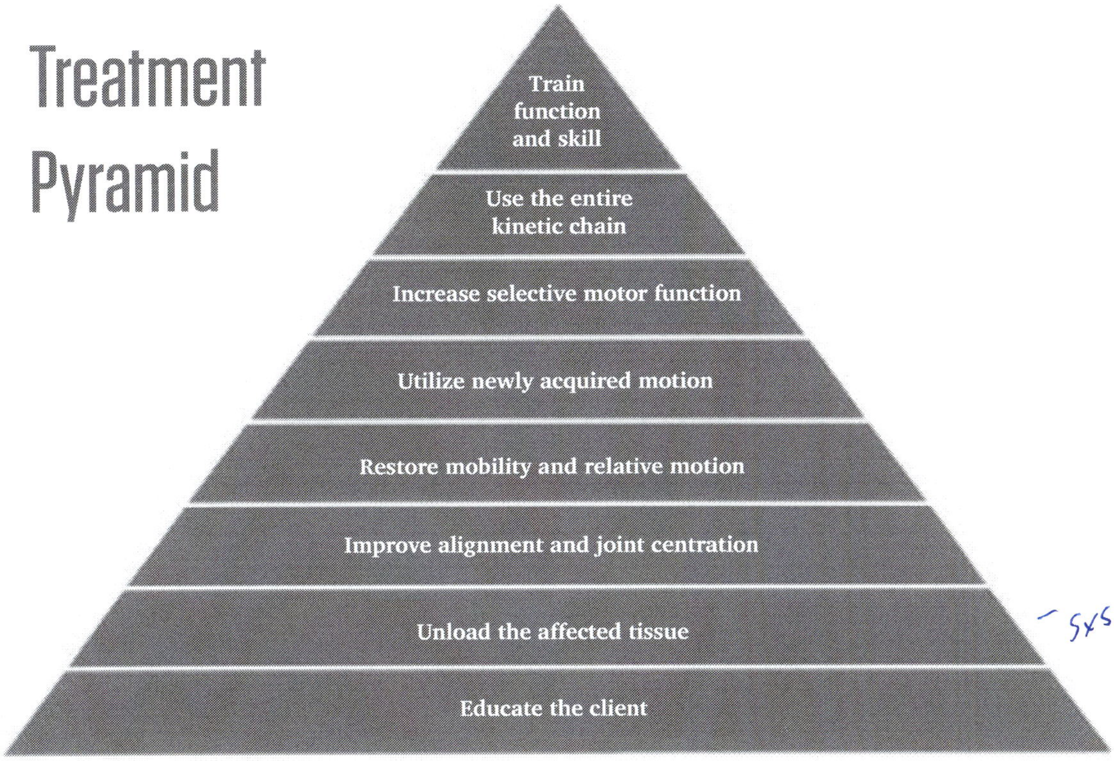
Train function and skill
Use the entire kinetic chain
Increase selective motor function
Utilize newly acquired motion
Restore mobility and relative motion
Improve alignment and joint centration
Unload the affected tissue
Educate the client

Copyright © 2019 Dr. Jared Vagy DPT

Developed by Jared Vagy. Inspired by Clare Frank and Phil Page

The Athlete Movement System: Upper Quarter

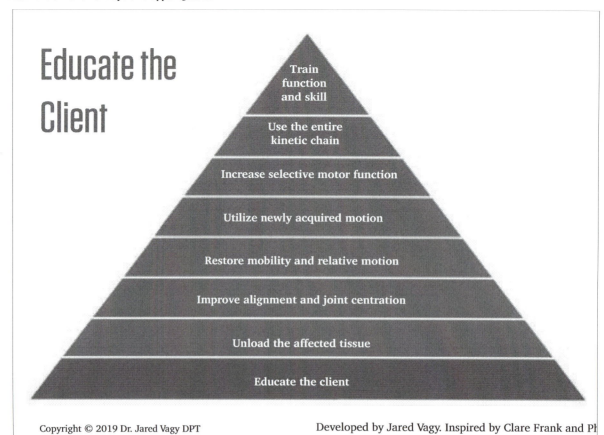

Educate the Client

- Train function and skill
- Use the entire kinetic chain
- Increase selective motor function
- Utilize newly acquired motion
- Restore mobility and relative motion
- Improve alignment and joint centration
- Unload the affected tissue
- Educate the client

Copyright © 2019 Dr. Jared Vagy DPT   Developed by Jared Vagy. Inspired by Clare Frank and Ph

Laddered Questions and Answer Planting

Ask laddered questions to plant the answer in their head and make the idea theirs.

Poor Client Education	Good Client Education
You need to tighten your stomach muscles when you throw the Javelin to decrease your shoulder pain.	**Question 1:** Which phase of throwing aggravates your shoulder when you throw? **Answer 1:** The acceleration phase. **Question 2:** I put your arm in that same phase a few minutes ago with a javelin and resistance band. What did you feel? **Answer 2:** Pain in my shoulder. **Question 3:** I then had you tighten your stomach muscles in that same position. What happened? **Answer 3:** I had no pain. **Question 4:** What do you think will help you get rid of your pain? **Answer 4:** I need to tighten my stomach muscles when I throw.

Copyright © 2019 Dr. Jared Vagy DPT

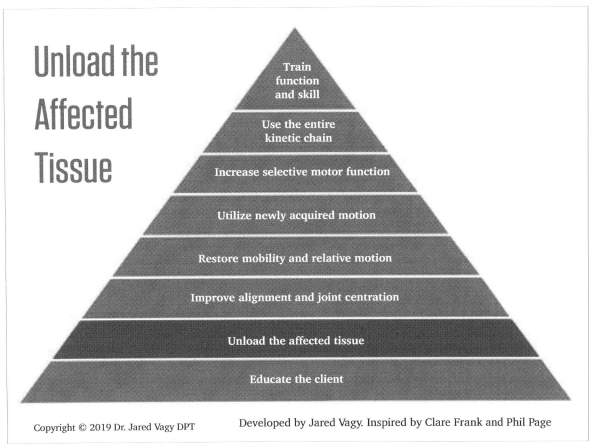

Unload the Affected Tissue

- Train function and skill
- Use the entire kinetic chain
- Increase selective motor function
- Utilize newly acquired motion
- Restore mobility and relative motion
- Improve alignment and joint centration
- Unload the affected tissue
- Educate the client

Copyright © 2019 Dr. Jared Vagy DPT   Developed by Jared Vagy. Inspired by Clare Frank and Phil Page

Examples of Unloading

Rigid Strap Tape

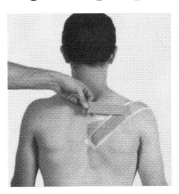

Promote scapular posterior tipping and lateral rotation

Kinesiology Tape

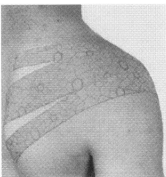

Inhibit anterior glide and medial rotation of the humerus

Pillows

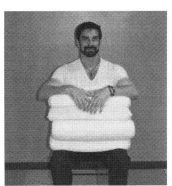

Prevent excessive scapular depression

Copyright © 2019 Dr. Jared Vagy DPT

Improve Alignment and Joint Centration

- Train function and skill
- Use the entire kinetic chain
- Increase selective motor function
- Utilize newly acquired motion
- Restore mobility and relative motion
- Improve alignment and joint centration
- Unload the affected tissue
- Educate the client

Copyright © 2019 Dr. Jared Vagy DPT   Developed by Jared Vagy. Inspired by Clare Frank and Phil Page

Research: Mechanisms of Joint Centration

- The joint force at end-range positions was more anteriorly directed than at mid-range. This indicates that its contribution to glenohumeral joint stability was diminished.
- In end-range positions, simulated increases in rotator cuff muscle forces improved stability whereas increases in deltoid or pectoralis major muscle forces decreased stability.

Increased rotator cuff function at end ranges improves joint stability.

Labriola, Joanne E., et al. JOSAES.14.1 (2005): S32-S38.

Joint Centration

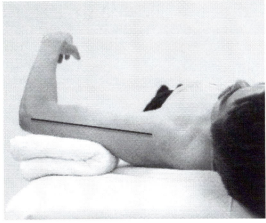
Centrated Joint

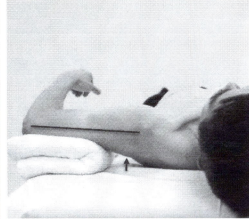
Non-centrated Joint
(anterior glide)

Joint Centration

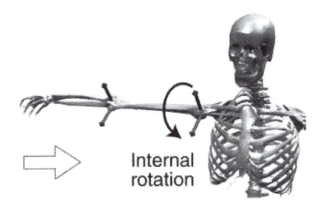
Internal rotation

When to use:
- Failed joint centration testing

What it does:
- Increases range of motion and motor control of the glenohumeral joint

Glenohumeral Joint Centration

How to perform:
- Pre-position patient in neutral humeral position
- Patient performs humeral medial rotation without compensation
- Use patient's hand as an initial tactile cue

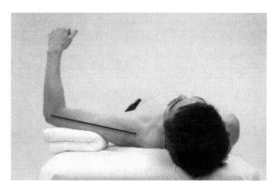
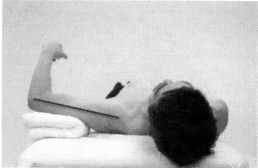

Summary

> Review joint centration as an assessment and treatment

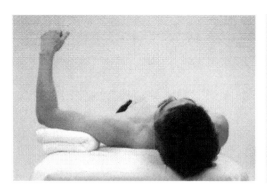
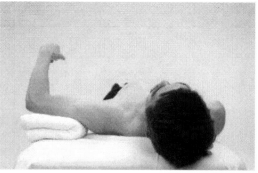

The Athlete Movement System: Upper Quarter

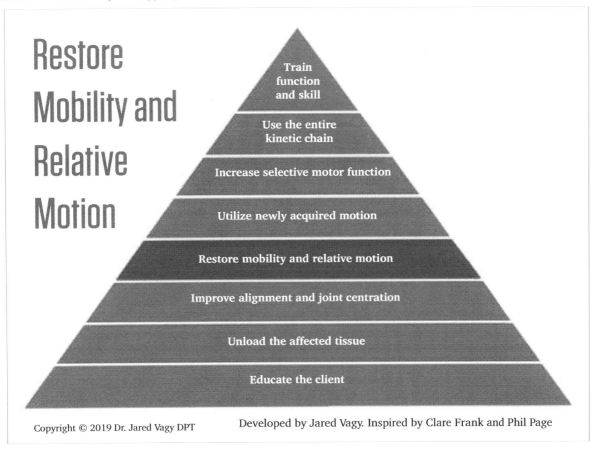

What is Relative Flexibility?

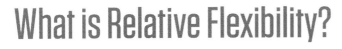

Short Latissimus Dorsi muscle

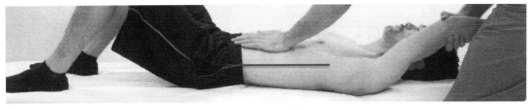

Relative stiffness of the Latissimus Dorsi muscle

Copyright © 2019 Dr. Jared Vagy DPT

3 Ways to Address Relative Flexibility

1. Increase Muscle Length - *Lengthen the black band*
- Soft Tissue Mobilization
- Stretching

2. Increase Intramuscular Stiffness - *Make the yellow band black*
- Stabilize the less stiff region while moving the stiffer region

3. Decrease Intramuscular Stiffness - *Make the black band yellow*
- Post Isometric Relaxation
- Gravity Induced Inhibition

Copyright © 2019 Dr. Jared Vagy DPT

1. Increase Muscle Length

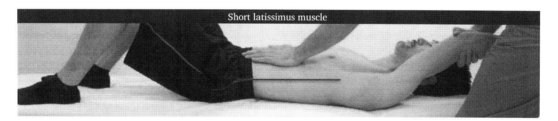
Short latissimus muscle

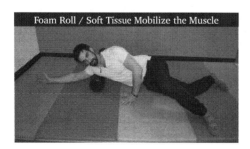
Foam Roll / Soft Tissue Mobilize the Muscle

OR

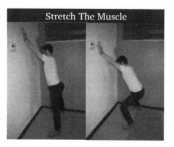
Stretch The Muscle

Copyright © 2019 Dr. Jared Vagy DPT

2. Increase Intramuscular Stiffness

Relative stiffness of Latissimus muscle vs lumbar spine

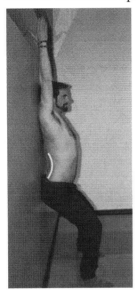

Corrected with increasing the stiffness of the abdominals

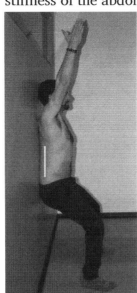

Copyright © 2019 Dr. Jared Vagy DPT

2. Decrease Intramuscular Stiffness

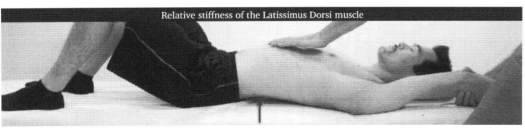

Relative stiffness of the Latissimus Dorsi muscle

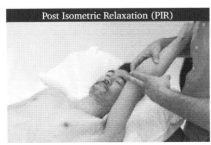

Post Isometric Relaxation (PIR)

OR

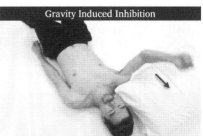

Gravity Induced Inhibition

Copyright © 2019 Dr. Jared Vagy DPT

Post Isometric Relaxation (PIR)

When to use:
- Hypertonicity and increased tissue tension in a muscle

What it does:
- The theory is that by using minimal resistance, specific fibers are activated and then inhibited. This is not a stretch.

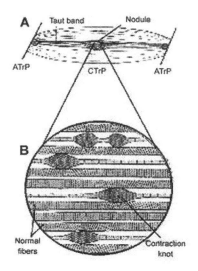

PIR of Latissimus Dorsi

How to perform:
- Slowly lengthen a muscle to first barrier.
- Patient pushes against you gently (10-20%).
- Patient hold contraction for 3-5 seconds.
- Take up slack to new barrier upon exhalation.
- Repeat 3-5 times.

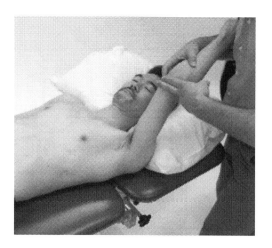

Gravity Induced Inhibition

When to use:
- Hypertonicity and increased tissue tension in a muscle throughout movement. For example, the inability to "let go."

What it does:
- The theory is that you can use gravity to train muscle inhibition by decreasing the muscular demand.

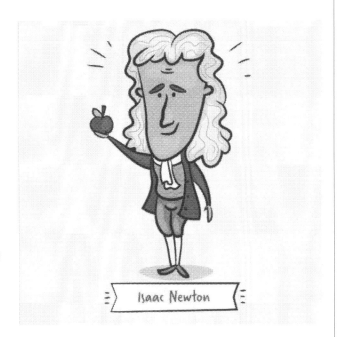

Gravity Induced Inhibition of Lats

How to perform:
- Slowly have the patient move the limb into the desired position of first muscle resistance.
- Give the cue "drop your arm"
- Patient then allows gravity to move their arm into an end range position.
- Repeat at least 150 times.

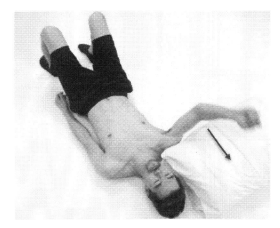

Wilde et al Res Q Exerc Sport 2005, Sherwood Res Q Exerc Sport 1996, and Douvis Percept Motor Skill 2005

Gravity Induced Inhibition of Lats

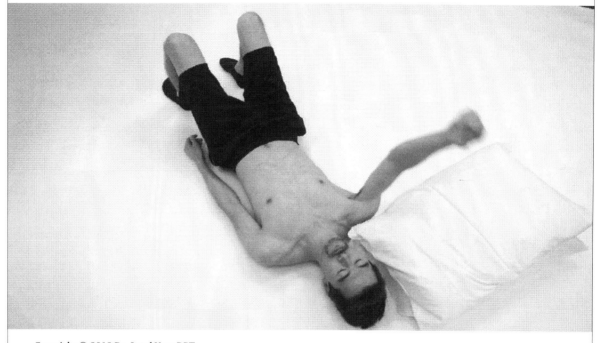

Copyright © 2019 Dr. Jared Vagy DPT

Summary

Review Lat muscle length test
Abdominal activation with arm raise
Post-Isometric Relaxation of Lat
Gravity induced inhibition of Lat

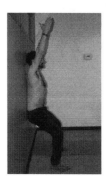 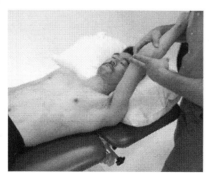 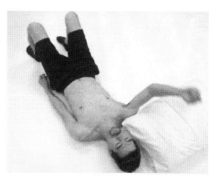

Copyright © 2019 Dr. Jared Vagy DPT

The Athlete Movement System: Upper Quarter

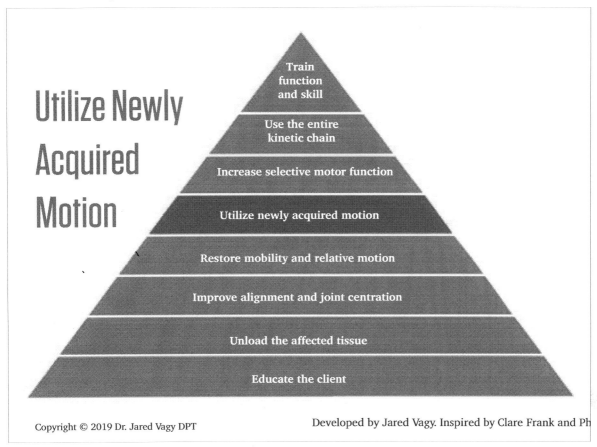

Research: Manipulation

- 21 Subjects with unilateral shoulder pain were deemed appropriate for upper thoracic spine manipulation.
- Outcome measures were shoulder pain (VAS) and AROM
- Measures were taken at evaluation and immediately after thrust manipulation
- No follow up

Significant decreases in pain rating and increases in range of motion immediately after manipulation

Strunce JB, cJ, Boyles RE, Young BA. The immediate effects of thoracic spine and rib manipulation on subjects with primary complaints of shoulder pain. *Journal of Manual and Manipulative Therapy.* 2009 (17:4) 230-236

Research: Mobilization and Exercise

- Two groups.
  - Group 1: Spinal manipulative therapy and exercise group.
  - Group 2: Spinal manipulative therapy.
- The spinal manipulative therapy and exercise group showed greater gains in all measures of strength, endurance, and range of motion than the spinal manipulation group.

The use of strengthening exercise in combination with spinal manipulation appears to be more beneficial to patients with chronic neck pain than the use of spinal manipulation alone.

Bronfort, Gert, et al. "A randomized clinical trial of exercise and spinal manipulation for patients with chronic neck pain." *Spine* 26.7 (2001): 788-797.

Utilize Motion Example 1: Clinical Findings

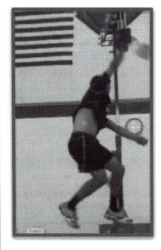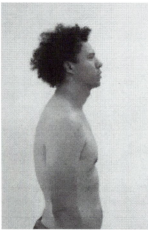

Complaint:
- Shoulder pain

Critical Event:
- Acceleration/ball contact phase of volleyball spike

Targeted Impairment:
- Thoracic spine hypomobility

Utilize Motion Example 1: Treatment

When to use:
- Directly after a mobilization technique.

What it does:
- Performed directly after mobilization techniques to utilize the newly acquired motion.

Step 1   Step 2   Step 3

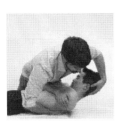 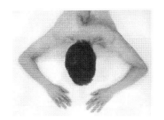 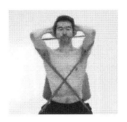

Copyright © 2019 Dr. Jared Vagy DPT

Step 1

Thoracic Spine Manipulation
- Apply prone or supine manipulation to thoracic spine

Prone PA
- Apply prone PA to thoracic spine unilateral or central

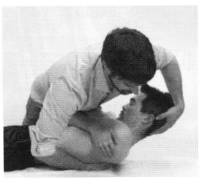   Or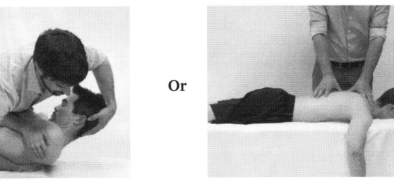

Copyright © 2019 Dr. Jared Vagy DPT

Step 2

Prone Deep Neck Flexion Thoracic Mobilization
- Place UE and LE in sport specific position.
- Therapist's thumb is placed below desired segment on the thoracic spine as patient lifts head.

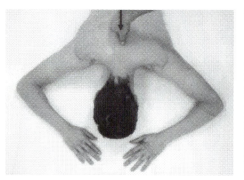 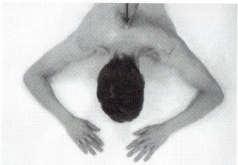

Step 2

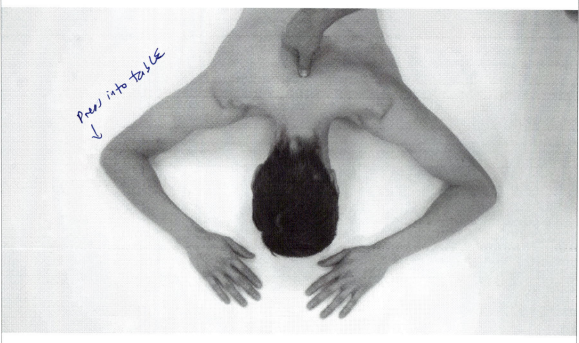

press into table

Step 3

Best for upper t/s

Seated Resisted Thoracic Extension
- Utilize a resistance band to apply resistance into thoracic extension.

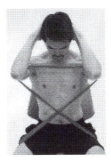 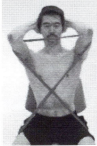 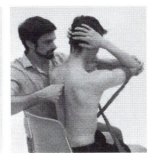 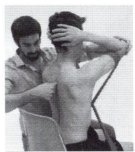

abduct into band can stabilize the L/s & prevent excessive lordosis

Step 3

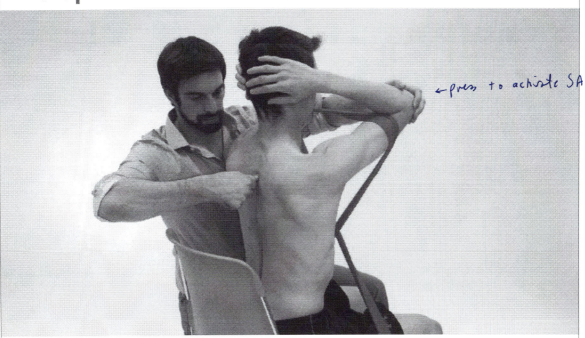

← press to activate SA

Summary

Hypomobile T/S
T/S accessory assessment
Mobilization or manipulation of thoracic spine
Deep neck flexion with thoracic pressure
Seated band wrap thoracic extension

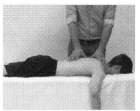 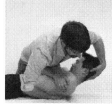 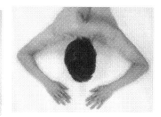 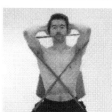

Utilize Motion Example 2: Clinical Findings

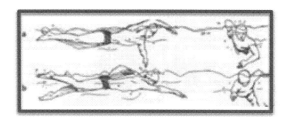

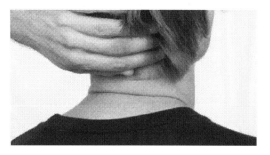

Complaint:
- Neck pain

Critical Event:
- Early pull through of freestyle swim stroke

Targeted Impairment:
- Short Levator Scapula

Utilize Motion Example 2: Treatment

When to use:
- Directly after a mobilization technique.

What it does:
- Performed directly after mobilization techniques to utilize the newly acquired motion.

Step 1	Step 2	Step 3
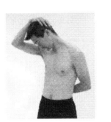	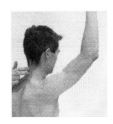	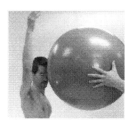

Step 1

Levator Stretch:
- Perform a manual or have the patient perform a self levator scapula stretch.

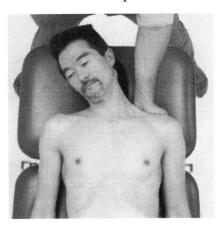 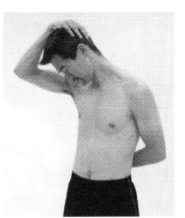

Step 2

Deep Neck Flexion with Arm Raise:
- Patient performs standing chin tuck
- Patient then flexes their shoulder
- No movement should occur in the cervical spine
  - Alternate position can be quadruped

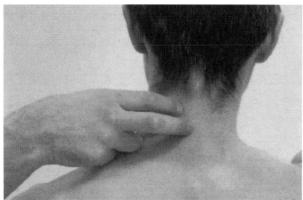
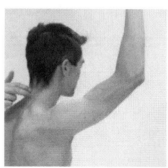

Copyright © 2019 Dr. Jared Vagy DPT

Step 3

Head Turn Ball Press with Arm Raise:
- Press your forehead into a ball on the wall as you raise your hand in the air

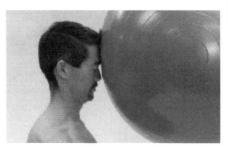
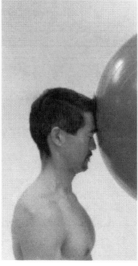
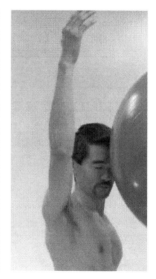

Copyright © 2019 Dr. Jared Vagy DPT

Step 3

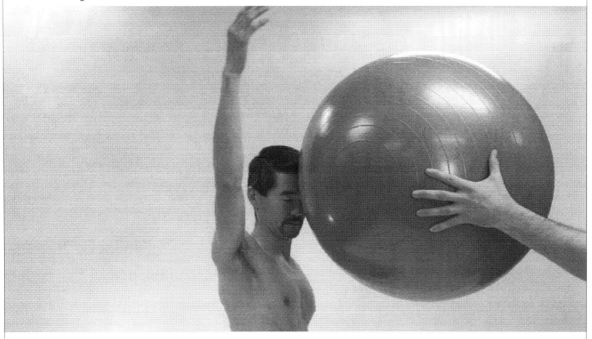

Summary

Short Levator Scap
Levator muscle length assessment
Levator stretch
Deep neck flexion with arm raise
Head turn ball press with arm raise

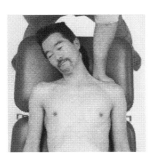 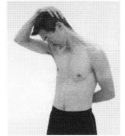 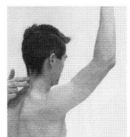 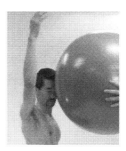

Utilize Motion Example 3: Clinical Findings

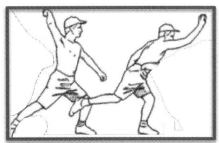

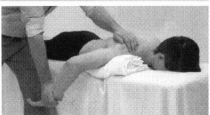

Complaint:
- Shoulder pain

Critical Event:
- Arm acceleration after late cocking

Targeted Impairment:
- Decreased glenohumeral medial rotation

Copyright © 2019 Dr. Jared Vagy DPT

Utilize Motion Example 3: Treatment

When to use:
- Directly after a mobilization technique.

What it does:
- Performed directly after mobilization techniques to utilize the newly acquired motion.

Step 1   Step 2   Step 3

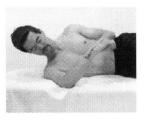 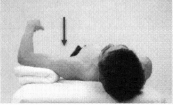 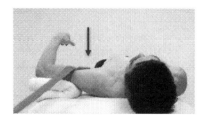

Copyright © 2019 Dr. Jared Vagy DPT

Step 1

Sleeper Stretch

- Patient performs side lying medial rotation stretch.

- Rotate your torso away from arm as you press your arm downward into medial rotation and maintain posterior glide of the humeral head.

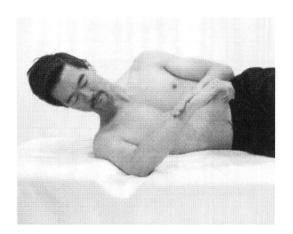

Copyright © 2019 Dr. Jared Vagy DPT

Step 2

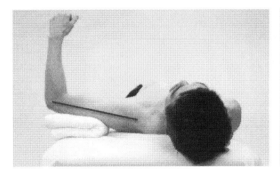 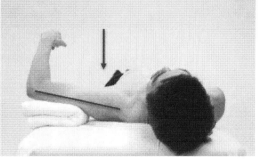

Glenohumeral Joint Centration

- Support the humerus with a folded towel.
- Rotate the humerus into medial rotation while maintaining posterior glide of the humeral head into the back of the table.
- Return to the starting position.

Copyright © 2019 Dr. Jared Vagy DPT

Step 3

Joint Centration with Rotation

- Support your humerus with a folded towel.
- Wrap a CLX band around your humerus (see wrapping instructions on the next page) so that it resists medial rotation and have a therapist hold the band or fixate it to a stationary object.
- Rotate the humerus into medial rotation while maintaining posterior glide of the humeral head into the back of the table.
- Return to the starting position.

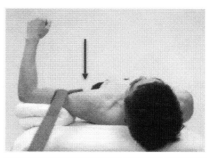
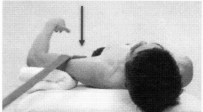

Copyright © 2019 Dr. Jared Vagy DPT

Joint Centration with Rotation

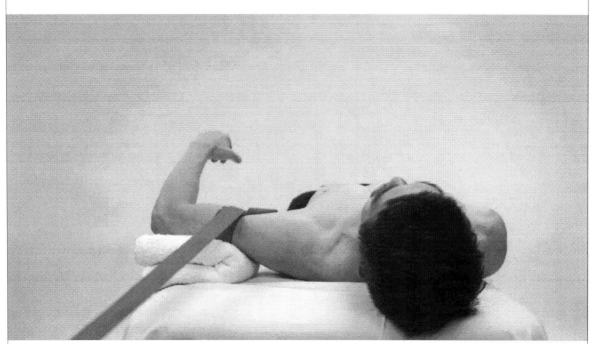

Copyright © 2019 Dr. Jared Vagy DPT

Step 3

How to wrap the band to resist humeral medial rotation:

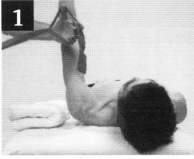
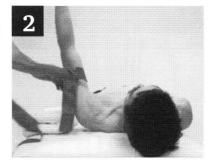
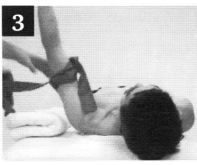
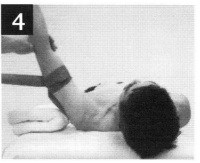

Copyright © 2019 Dr. Jared Vagy DPT

Step 3

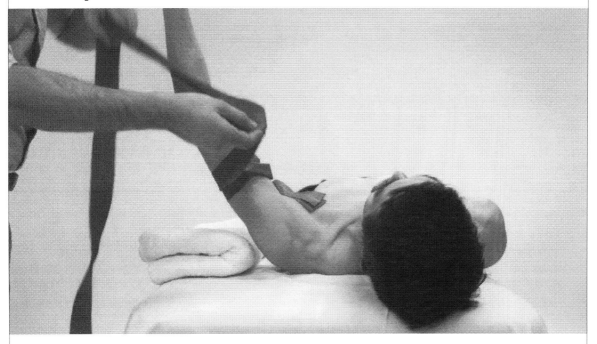

Copyright © 2019 Dr. Jared Vagy DPT

Why Choose One Over The Other?

Supine Resisted Medial Rotation:
* Band wrapped around humerus

Supine Resisted Medial Rotation:
* Band wrapped around hand

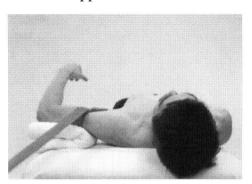
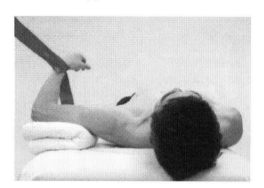

Summary

Decreased Glenohumeral Medial Rotation
Decreased AROM and PROM of medial rotation
Modified sleeper stretch
Joint centration
Medial rotations with resistance

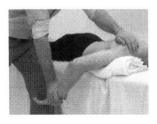 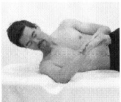 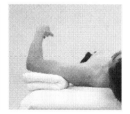 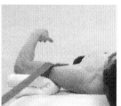

The Athlete Movement System: Upper Quarter

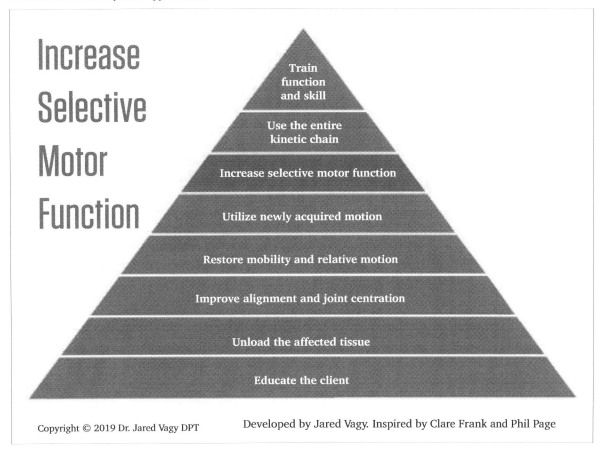

Copyright © 2019 Dr. Jared Vagy DPT   Developed by Jared Vagy. Inspired by Clare Frank and Phil Page

How to Target the Muscle

Muscular Facilitation   **Reflexive Activation**   **Vectors**

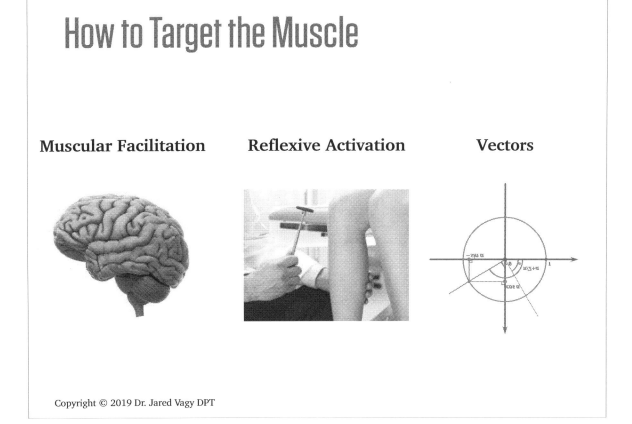

Copyright © 2019 Dr. Jared Vagy DPT

Muscular Facilitation

Muscular Facilitation

When to use:
- Failed manual muscle test of impaired muscle

What it does:
- Increases the motor function of the muscle

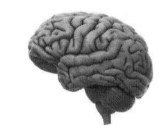
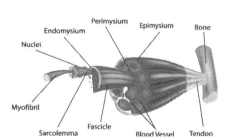

Muscular Facilitation of Mid Trap

How to perform:
- Patient is prone or quadruped.
- Shoulder is flexed and abducted to the desired position.
- Therapist presses thumb into medial scapular border at varied angles.
- Patient contracts into the thumb.
- Tapping the muscle can improve facilitation.

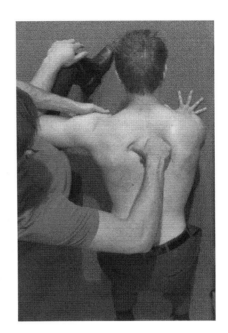

Reflexive Activation

Reflexive (Backdoor) Activation

- Designed to activate muscles as they function.

- Exercise happens automatically during movement without conscious control.

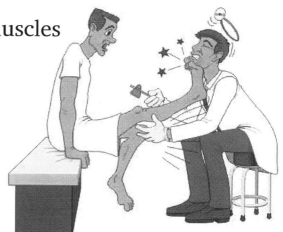

Copyright © 2019 Dr. Jared Vagy DPT

Reflexive Exercise for Deep Neck Flexors

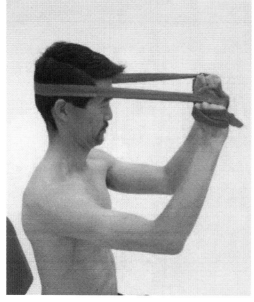

Deep Neck Flexors   **Sport Specific Deep Neck Flexors**

Copyright © 2019 Dr. Jared Vagy DPT

The Athlete Movement System: Upper Quarter

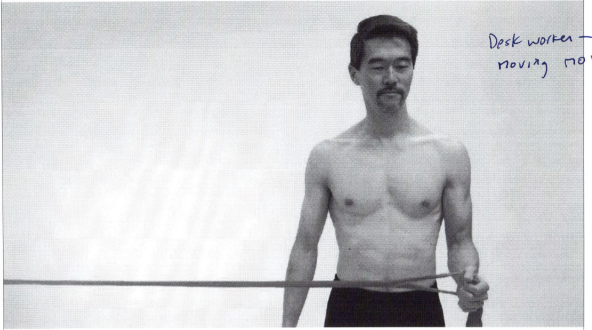

Desk worker — moving mouse

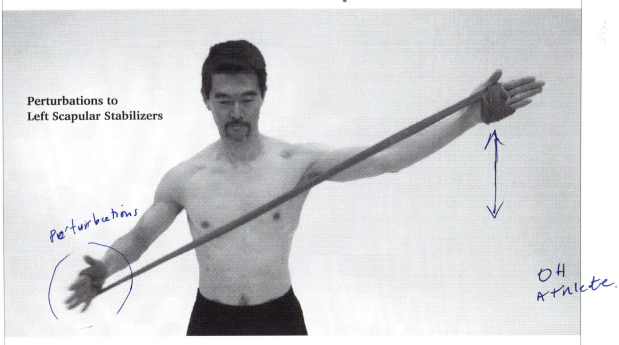

OH Athlete

121

Vectors

- Direction of force towards or away from the muscle action.

- Vectors have two independent properties:
  - Magnitude
  - Direction

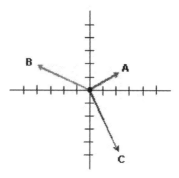
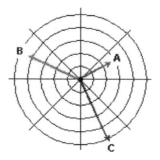

Vector Magnitude

- **Resistance is quantifiable**

TheraBand Color	Progressive Increase at 100%	Band or Tube Elongation 100% (pounds)	200% (pounds)
Tan	-	2.4	3.4
Yellow	25%	3	4.2
Red	25%	3.7	5.2
Green	25%	4.6	6.4
Blue	25%	5.8	8.1
Black	25%	7.3	10.2
Silver	40%	10.2	14.8
Gold	40%	14.2	20.6

Percentage elongation = [(final − resting) / (resting)] X 100

Vector Direction

Vector of assistance *w/ Body bouncing*

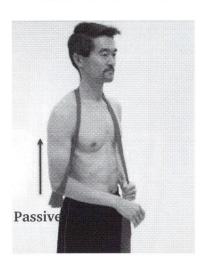

Passive

Vector of resistance

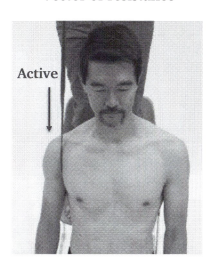

Active

The Athlete Movement System: Upper Quarter

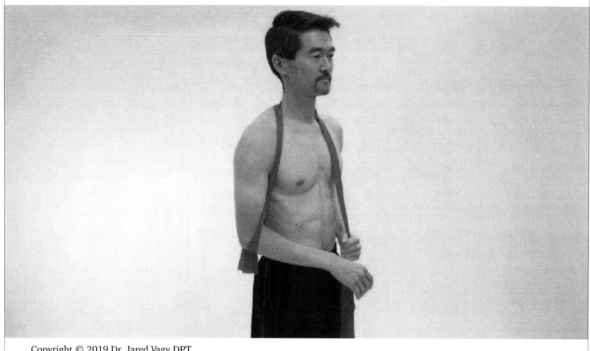

Vector of Assistance

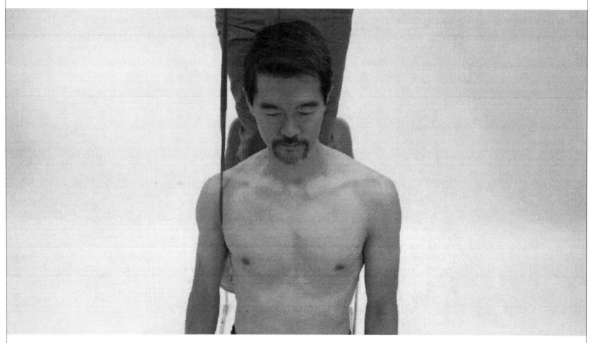

Vector of Resistance

Dual Vector High Band

Vectors of assistance
- Scapular/humeral elevation

Vectors of resistance:
- Humeral lateral rotation

Vectors of resistance
- Scapular/humeral depression

Vectors of resistance:
- Humeral lateral rotation

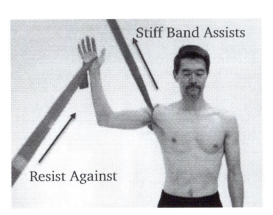
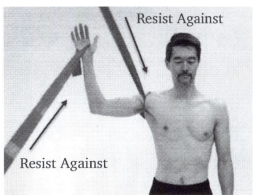

Dual Vector Low Band

Vectors of assistance
- Scapular/humeral depression

Vectors of resistance:
- Humeral lateral rotation — Thick STB

Vectors of resistance
- Scapular/humeral elevation

Vectors of resistance:
- Humeral lateral rotation

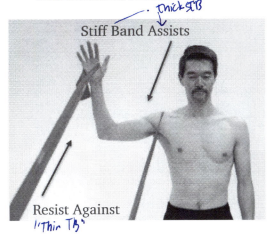
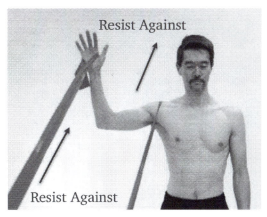

"Thin TB"

Dual Vector

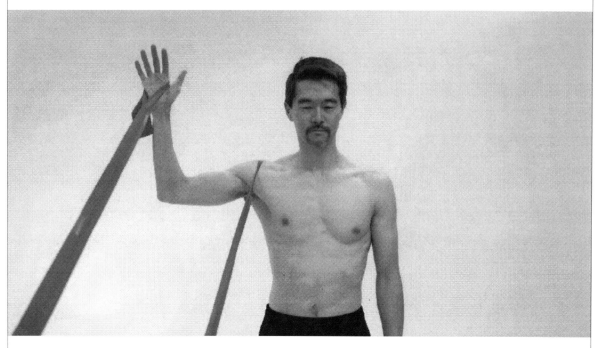

Summary

Muscular Facilitation	Muscle facilitation of Mid Trap Prone and quadruped
Reflexive Activation	Deep neck flexors Scapular stabilizers Rotator Cuff lateral rotators
Vectors	Vectors of assistance Vectors of resistance

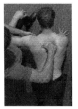 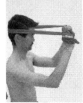 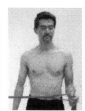 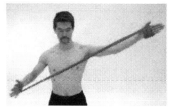 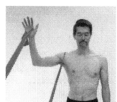

The Athlete Movement System: Upper Quarter

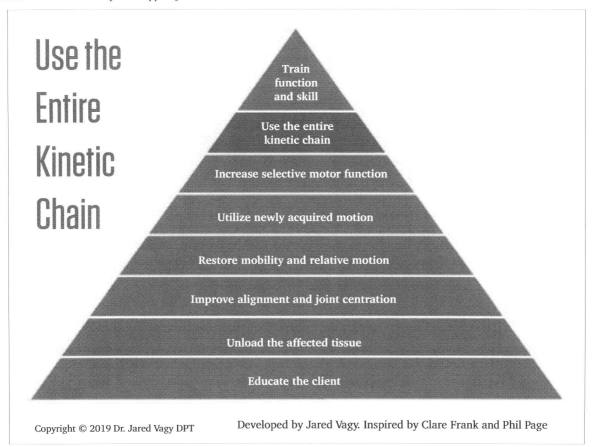

Use the Entire Kinetic Chain

- Train function and skill
- Use the entire kinetic chain
- Increase selective motor function
- Utilize newly acquired motion
- Restore mobility and relative motion
- Improve alignment and joint centration
- Unload the affected tissue
- Educate the client

Copyright © 2019 Dr. Jared Vagy DPT   Developed by Jared Vagy. Inspired by Clare Frank and Phil Page

Kinetic Chain

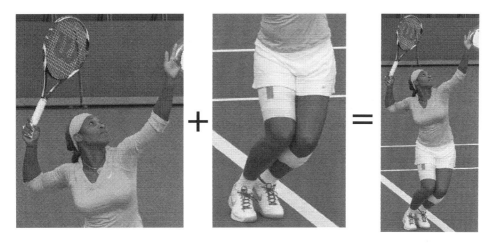

It is essential to treat the entire kinetic chain. If you don't analyze movement, you are missing a large piece of the puzzle.

Copyright © 2019 Dr. Jared Vagy DPT

Research: Regional Interdependence

- A patient with lateral epicondylagia and postural/functional scapular malpositioning.
- Interventions targeted at the scapula with both movement re-education and strengthening exercises.
- Improved middle and lower trapezius strength, scapular position and symptoms. DASH questionnaire improved from 44.2 at the initial evaluation to 0.

Treat what appears to be causing the dysfunction rather than focus solely on treatment of symptoms. This often requires treating an adjacent, or even remote area.

[CASE REPORT]

Middle and Lower Trapezius Strengthening for the Management of Lateral Epicondylalgia: A Case Report

Bhatt, Jiten B., et al. JOSPT, 43.11 (2013): 841-847.

How to Target the Kinetic Chain

Neuromuscular Chains *(Janda)*

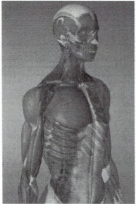
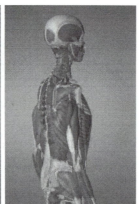

Muscle Slings

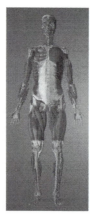
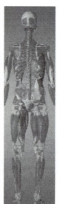
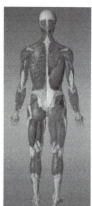

The Athlete Movement System: Upper Quarter

Neuromuscular Chains

Neuromuscular Chains Janda 1987, Frank 2015

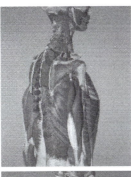
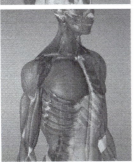

Tonic System	Phasic System
Older system	Younger system
Flexor system	Extensor system
Tend to shorten	Tend to lengthen/atrophy
Overactivation	Delayed activation
Dominate • Intrauterine & early infancy • Sedentarism and deconditioning • Old age and injury	Recessive • Requires higher CNS control • Easily inhibited

The Athlete Movement System: Upper Quarter

Tonic Muscle Chain

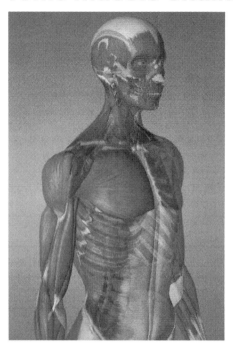

Muscles Involved
- Pec major/minor
- Upper trapezius
- Levator scapula
- SCM / scalenes
- Suboccipitals
- Upper limb flexors
- Thoracolumbar extensors

Copyright © 2017 Dr. Jared Vagy

Janda 1987, Frank 2015

Phasic Muscle Chain

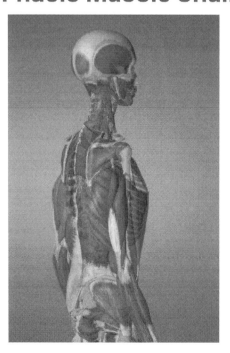

Muscles Involved
- Serratus anterior
- Mid/lower traps
- Rhomboids
- Deep neck flexors
- Upper limb extensors

Copyright © 2017 Dr. Jared Vagy

Janda 1987, Frank 2015

Apply to Sport

Tonic Chain:
- Shoulder and elbow flexion
- Shoulder horizontal adduction
- Shoulder medial rotation
- Scapular abduction
- Forearm pronation

Phasic Chain:
- Shoulder and elbow extension
- Shoulder horizontal abduction
- Shoulder lateral rotation
- Scapular adduction
- Forearm supination

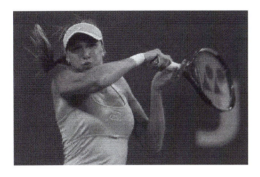
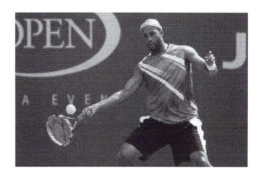

Copyright © 2017 Dr. Jared Vagy

Adapted from Frank, Movement Links 2015

Neuromuscular Chains Quadruped

Brueger exercises?

Tonic:
- Shoulder and elbow flexion
- Shoulder horizontal adduction
- Shoulder medial rotation
- Scapular abduction
- Forearm pronation

Phasic Chain:
- Shoulder and elbow extension
- Shoulder horizontal abduction
- Shoulder lateral rotation
- Scapular adduction
- Forearm supination

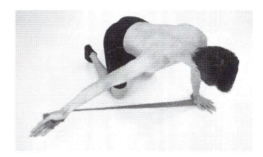

Targets the underutilized phasic chain in quadruped

Copyright © 2017 Dr. Jared Vagy

Neuromuscular Chains Sitting

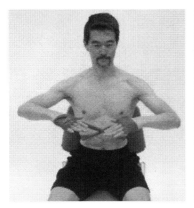
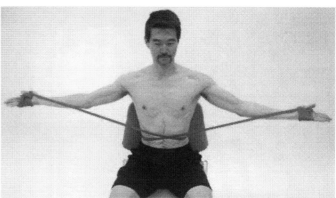

Targets the underutilized phasic chain in sitting

Neuromuscular Chains Standing

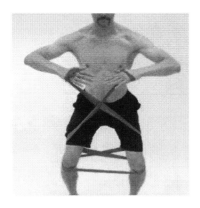
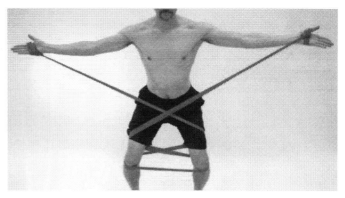

Targets the underutilized phasic chain in standing

Summary

Phases Chain Exercises	Phasic pattern quadruped Phasic pattern seated Phasic pattern standing

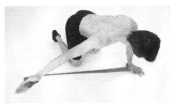 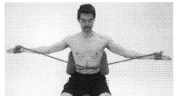 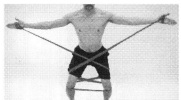

Muscle Slings

Muscle Slings

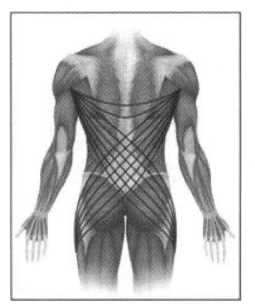
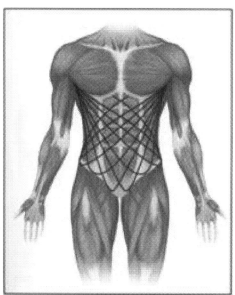

Muscle Slings

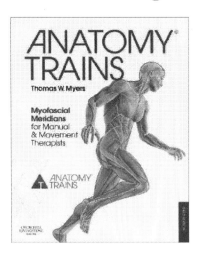
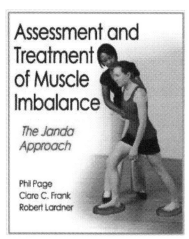

- Muscles are interconnected through the fascial system.
- Slings, chains, trains, and loops provide movement and stabilization across multiple joints.

Upper Extremity Flexor Sling

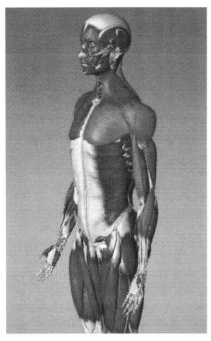

- Pectoralis major
- Anterior deltoid
- Trapezius
- Biceps
- Wrist and finger flexors

Copyright © 2017 Dr. Jared Vagy

Upper Extremity Extensor Sling

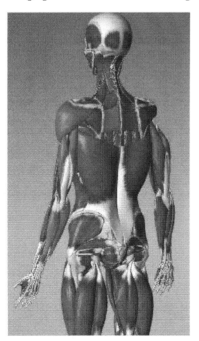

- Rhomboids
- Posterior deltoid
- Triceps
- Wrist and finger extensors

Copyright © 2017 Dr. Jared Vagy

Anterior Trunk Sling

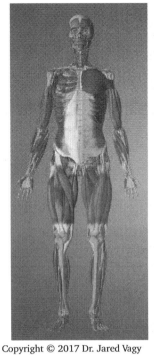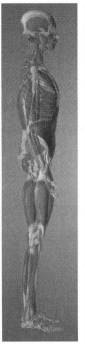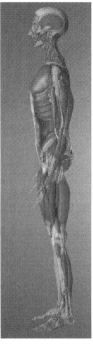

- Ipsilateral biceps and pectoralis major
- Contralateral internal oblique, hip abductors, sartorius and quadriceps

Anterior Trunk Sling

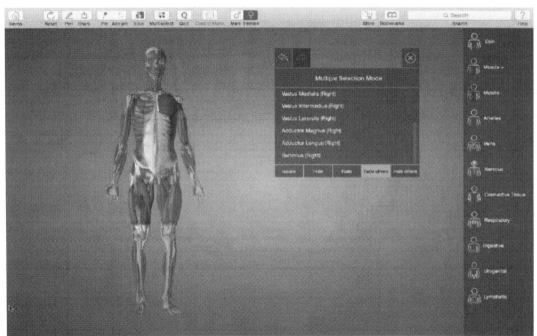

Anterior Trunk Sling Exercise Short Lever

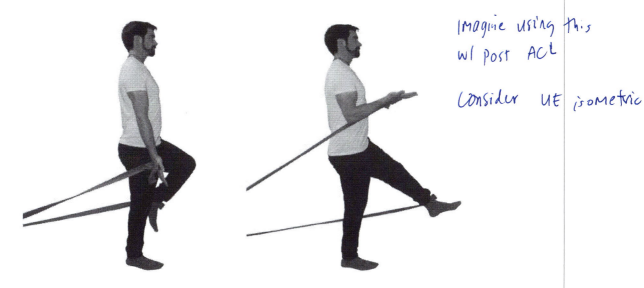

Imagine using this w/ post ACL

Consider UE isometric

Utilizes the knee extensors to facilitate the elbow flexors

Copyright © 2019 Dr. Jared Vagy DPT

Anterior Trunk Sling Exercise Short Lever

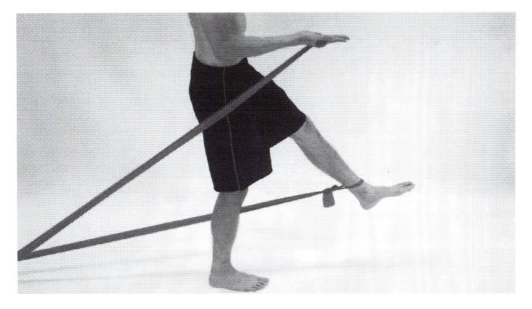

Utilizes the knee extensors to facilitate the elbow flexors

Copyright © 2019 Dr. Jared Vagy DPT

Anterior Trunk Sling Exercise Long Lever

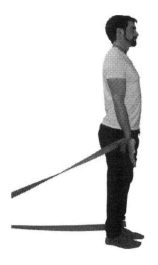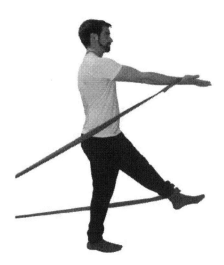

Utilizes the femoral flexors to facilitate the humeral flexors

Anterior Trunk Sling Exercise 1

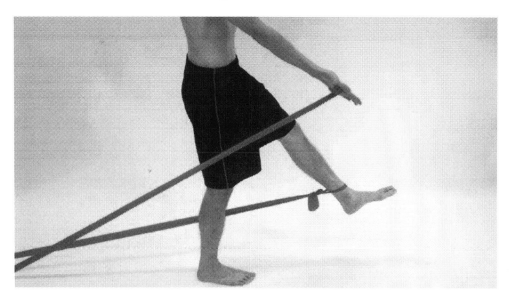

Utilizes the knee extensors to facilitate the elbow flexors

Posterior Trunk Sling

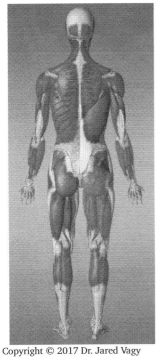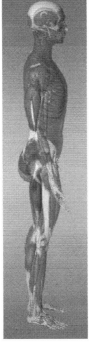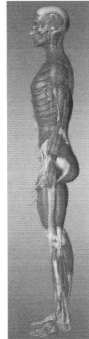

- Ipsilateral triceps and latissimus dorsi
- Contralateral thoracolumbar fascia, gluteus maximus and hamstrings

Posterior Trunk Sling

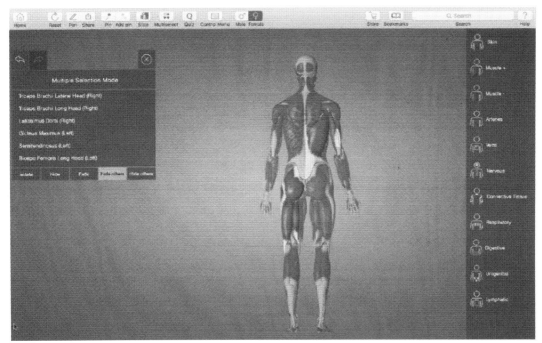

Posterior Trunk Sling Exercise Short Lever

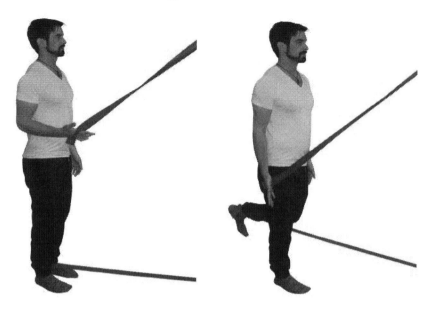

Utilizes the knee flexors to facilitate the elbow extensors

Copyright © 2019 Dr. Jared Vagy DPT

Posterior Trunk Sling Exercise Short Lever

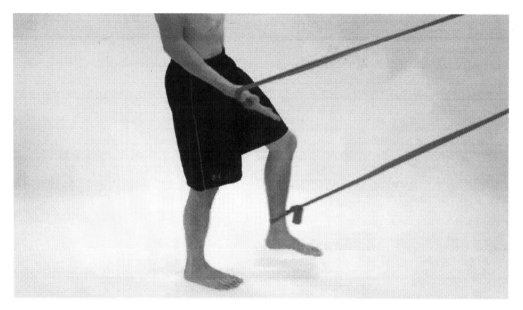

Utilizes the knee flexors to facilitate the elbow extensors

Copyright © 2019 Dr. Jared Vagy DPT

Posterior Trunk Sling Exercise Long Lever

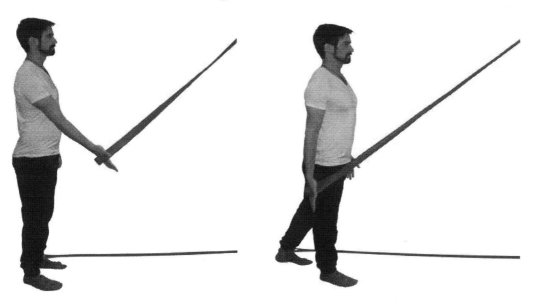

Utilizes the femoral extensors to facilitate the humeral extensors

Copyright © 2019 Dr. Jared Vagy DPT

Posterior Trunk Sling Exercise Long Lever

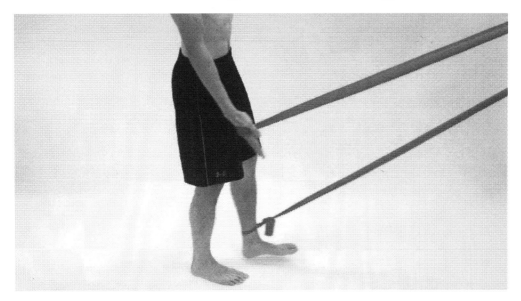

Utilizes the femoral extensors to facilitate the humeral extensors

Copyright © 2019 Dr. Jared Vagy DPT

Summary

Slings	Anterior trunk sling short lever Anterior trunk sling long lever Posterior trunk sling short lever Posterior trunk sling lever

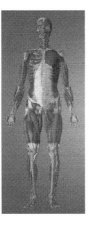
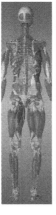
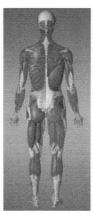

Copyright © 2019 Dr. Jared Vagy DPT

Spiral Trunk Sling

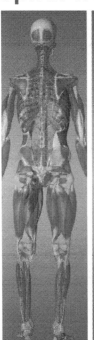
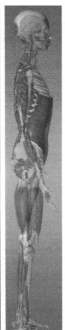
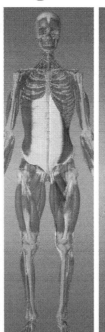
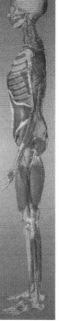

- Ipsilateral rhomboids, serratus anterior and external oblique
- Contralateral internal oblique and hip adductors

Copyright © 2017 Dr. Jared Vagy

Spiral Trunk Sling

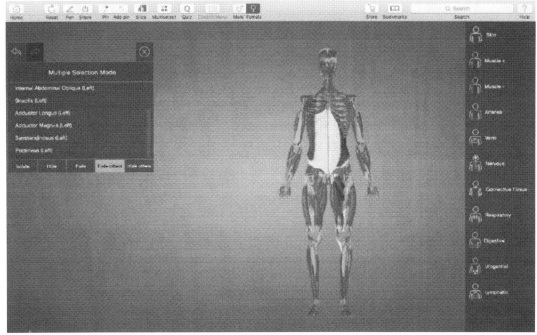

Strap Exercise Video

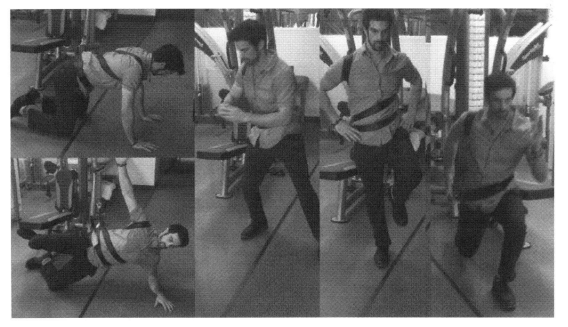

Summary

Stap Exercises
Level 1: Quadruped UE and LE raises
Level 2: Side plank with and without clamshell
Level 3: Loaded squat
Level 4: Single leg balance rotational stability
Level 5: Lunge

Copyright © 2019 Dr. Jared Vagy DPT

Research: Pelvic Rotational Stability

- The relationship of the gluteals to pelvis kinematics during baseball pitching.
- Gluteus maximus activity was related to the rate of axial pelvis rotation.
- Previous studies have shown pitchers with difficulty controlling the rate of trunk rotation may increase their risks for injury.

Indicates that during the baseball pitch, there is a need for greater control of gluteal activation throughout the pitching motion.

Oliver et al. J Strength Cond Res; 24.11 (2010): 3015-3022.

Additional Slings

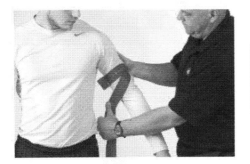

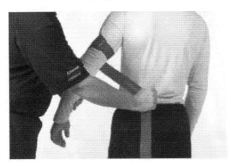

Hip lateral rotators with throwing

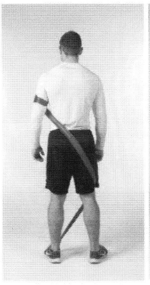
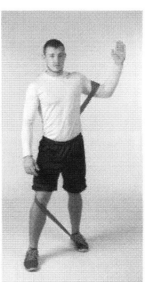

Additional Slings

Scapular stabilizers, obliques, and multifidi with hitting

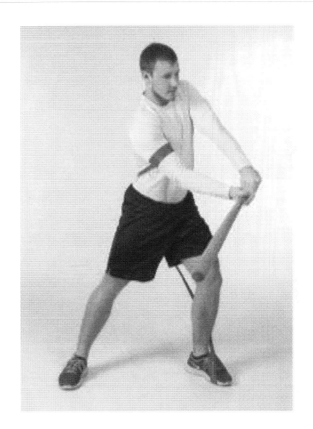

The Athlete Movement System: Upper Quarter

Summary

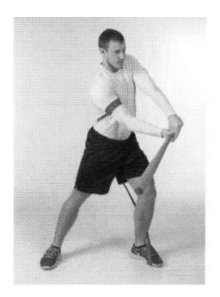
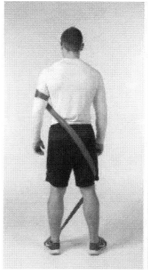
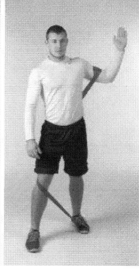

Swing functional sling with CLX   **Throw functional sling with CLX**

Copyright © 2019 Dr. Jared Vagy DPT

Train Function and Skill

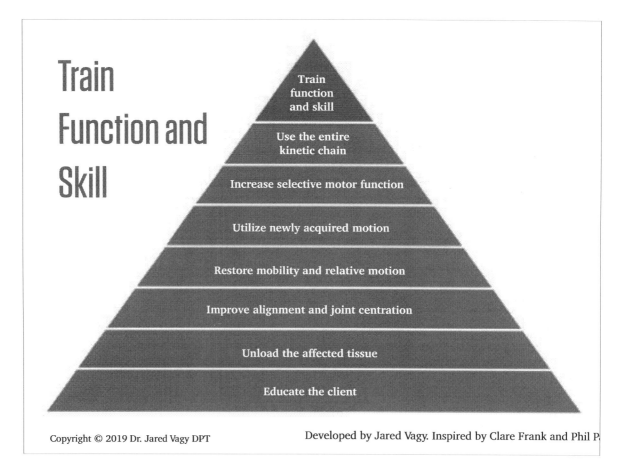

- Train function and skill
- Use the entire kinetic chain
- Increase selective motor function
- Utilize newly acquired motion
- Restore mobility and relative motion
- Improve alignment and joint centration
- Unload the affected tissue
- Educate the client

Copyright © 2019 Dr. Jared Vagy DPT   Developed by Jared Vagy. Inspired by Clare Frank and Phil P

The Athlete Movement System: Upper Quarter

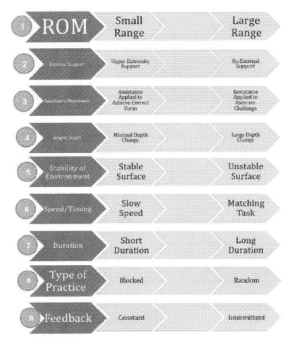

Copyright © 2019 Dr. Jared Vagy DPT

Swim

- Swimming (Freestyle)
  - Prone on exercise ball
    - Scapular retraction with theraband in early recovery phase
    - Scapular upward rotation and protraction with theraband in early pull-through phase

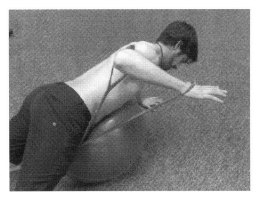 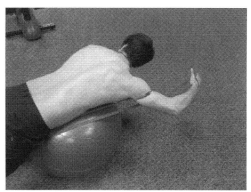

Copyright © 2019 Dr. Jared Vagy DPT

Tennis

- Backhand
  - Hip lateral rotation during wind up
  - Rotational stability of the oblique musculature

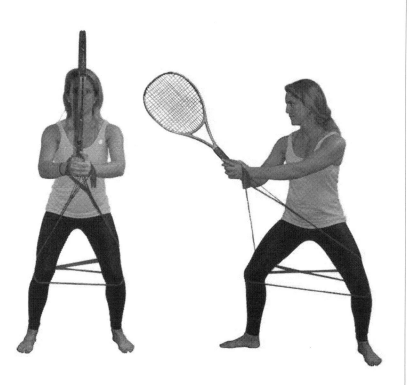

Copyright © 2019 Dr. Jared Vagy DPT

Baseball

- Throwing
  - Scapular stabilization at late cocking phase
  - Shoulder eccentric IR at acceleration phase
  - Scapular stabilization at deceleration phase

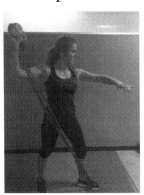 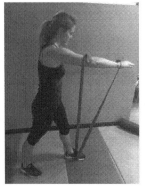 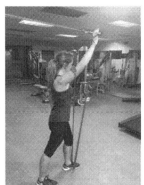

Copyright © 2019 Dr. Jared Vagy DPT

Volleyball

- Spike
  - Shoulder abduction/ER at ball contact (with theraband)

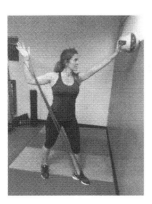 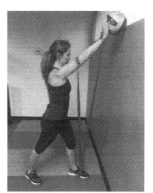

Climbing

Reverse Outside Flag
- Mirroring positions on the rock with sliders on the ground

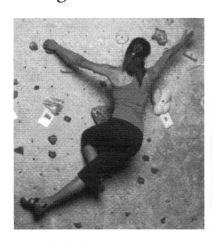 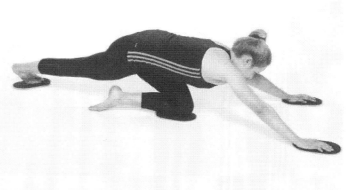

Research: Weight Bearing Exercise

- Analyzed prayer quadruped, quadruped arm raise, quadruped arm and leg raise, push-up, push-up feet elevated one-arm push-up.
- Each exercise progression had increased EMG activity of infraspinatus.

Alterations of weight-bearing exercises, by varying the amount of arm support and force, resulted in very different demands on the shoulder musculature.

Uhl, Tim L., et al. JOSPT. 33.3 (2003): 109-117.

Sliders

Slider Exercise Example

Flag

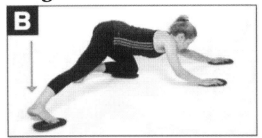

Reverse Outside Flag

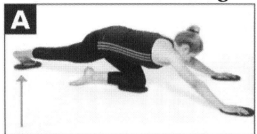

- Utilize weight bearing positions to add additional levels of muscle recruitment and stability.
- Try to mirror positions similar to sport to achieve full kinetic chain involvement .

Copyright © 2019 Dr. Jared Vagy DPT

Take Home Message

- Follow a the framework of a rehabilitation pyramid to sequence and organize your treatments.

- Utilize movement based treatment techniques of joint centration, post isometric relaxation, gravity induced inhibition to enhance your treatment results.

- Understand the concepts of muscular facilitation, reflexive activation, vectors, neuromuscular chains, muscle slings, and sport specific exercises that target the entire movement system and use them selectivity to achieve your desired results.

- Progress your treatments into sport specific skill by taking advantage of neuromuscular chains and muscle slings.

Copyright © 2019 Dr. Jared Vagy DPT

Made in the USA
San Bernardino, CA
03 March 2019